Endoscopy

Editor

MARYANN G. RADLINSKY

VETERINARY CLINICS OF NORTH AMERICA: SMALL ANIMAL PRACTICE

www.vetsmall.theclinics.com

January 2016 • Volume 46 • Number 1

ELSEVIER

1600 John F. Kennedy Boulevard • Suite 1800 • Philadelphia, Pennsylvania, 19103-2899

http://www.vetsmall.theclinics.com

**VETERINARY CLINICS OF NORTH AMERICA: SMALL ANIMAL PRACTICE Volume 46, Number 1
January 2016 ISSN 0195-5616, ISBN-13: 978-0-323-41476-0**

Editor: Patrick Manley

Developmental Editor: Meredith Clinton

Veterinary Clinics of North America: Small Animal Practice (ISSN 0195-5616) is published bimonthly by Elsevier Inc., 360 Park Avenue South, New York, NY 10010-1710. Months of issue are January, March, May, July, September, and November. Business and Editorial Offices: 1600 John F. Kennedy Blvd., Ste. 1800, Philadelphia, PA 19103-2899. Customer Service Office: 3251 Riverport Lane, Maryland Heights, MO 63043. Periodicals postage paid at New York, NY and additional mailing offices. Subscription prices are $310.00 per year (domestic individuals), $564.00 per year (domestic institutions), $100.00 per year (domestic students/residents), $410.00 per year (Canadian individuals), $701.00 per year (Canadian institutions), $455.00 per year (international individuals), $701.00 per year (international institutions), and $220.00 per year (international and Canadian students/residents). To receive student/resident rate, orders must be accompanied by name of affiliated institution, date of term, and the *signature* of program/residency coordinator on institution letterhead. Orders will be billed at individual rate until proof of status is received. Foreign air speed delivery is included in all *Clinics* subscription prices. All prices are subject to change without notice. **POSTMASTER:** Send address changes to *Veterinary Clinics of North America: Small Animal Practice*, Elsevier Health Sciences Division, Subscription Customer Service, 3251 Riverport Lane, Maryland Heights, MO 63043. Customer Service (orders, claims, online, change of address): Elsevier Periodicals Customer Service, Elsevier Health Sciences Division Subscription **Customer Service 3251 Riverport Lane Maryland Heights, MO 63043. Tel: 1-800-654-2452 (U.S. and Canada); 314-447-8871 (outside U.S. and Canada). Fax: 314-447-8029. E-mail: journalscustomerservice-usa@elsevier.com (for print support); journalsonlinesupport-usa@elsevier.com (for online support).**

Reprints. For copies of 100 or more of articles in this publication, please contact the Commercial Reprints Department, Elsevier Inc., 360 Park Avenue South, New York, NY 10010-1710. Tel.: 212-633-3874; Fax: 212-633-3820; E-mail: reprints@elsevier.com.

Veterinary Clinics of North America: Small Animal Practice is also published in Japanese by Inter Zoo Publishing Co., Ltd., Aoyama Crystal-Bldg 5F, 3-5-12 Kitaaoyama, Minato-ku, Tokyo 107-0061, Japan.

Veterinary Clinics of North America: Small Animal Practice is covered in *Current Contents/Agriculture, Biology and Environmental Sciences, Science Citation Index, ASCA, MEDLINE/PubMed (Index Medicus), Excerpta Medica,* and *BIOSIS.*

Contributors

EDITOR

MARYANN G. RADLINSKY, DVM, MS
Diplomate, American College of Veterinary Surgeons; Department of Small Animal Medicine and Surgery, College of Veterinary Medicine, The University of Georgia, Athens, Georgia

AUTHORS

MAKOTO ASAKAWA, BVSc
Diplomate, American College of Veterinary Anesthesia and Analgesia; Department of Clinical Sciences, Cornell University College of Veterinary Medicine, Ithaca, New York

ALLYSON C. BERENT, DVM
Diplomate, American College of Veterinary Internal Medicine; Director, Interventional Endoscopy Services, Department of Small Animal Internal Medicine, The Animal Medical Center, New York, New York

JOSEPH BRAD CASE, DVM, MS
Diplomate, American College of Veterinary Surgeons; Assistant Professor, Small Animal Surgery, College of Veterinary Medicine, University of Florida, Gainesville, Florida

BOEL A. FRANSSON, DVM, PhD
Diplomate, American College of Veterinary Surgeons; Associate Professor of Small Animal Surgery, Department of Veterinary Clinical Sciences, Washington State University, Pullman, Washington

JOHN C. HUHN, DVM, MS
Medical Director, Animal Health, Medtronic, Salem, Connecticut

ANANT RADHAKRISHNAN, DVM
Diplomate, American College of Veterinary Internal Medicine; Department of Internal Medicine, Bluegrass Veterinary Specialists + Animal Emergency, Lexington, Kentucky

MARYANN G. RADLINSKY, DVM, MS
Diplomate, American College of Veterinary Surgeons; Department of Small Animal Medicine and Surgery, College of Veterinary Medicine, The University of Georgia, Athens, Georgia

JEFFREY J. RUNGE, DVM
Diplomate, American College of Veterinary Surgeons; Assistant Professor of Minimally Invasive Surgery, Section of Surgery, Department of Clinical Studies, School of Veterinary Medicine, University of Pennsylvania, Philadelphia, Pennsylvania

MICHELE A. STEFFEY, DVM
Diplomate, American College of Veterinary Surgeons; Associate Professor of Small Animal Surgery, Department of Surgical and Radiological Sciences, School of Veterinary Medicine, University of California Davis, Davis, California

CHLOE WORMSER, VMD
Section of Surgery, Department of Clinical Studies, School of Veterinary Medicine, University of Pennsylvania, Philadelphia, Pennsylvania

Contents

Veterinarians interested in adding minimally invasive surgery (MIS) to their surgical repertoire need a distinct set of skills. These MIS skills do not transfer from open surgery; they require specific training. Training based solely on practice in live patients becomes limited and inconsistent. In addition, ethical and financial issues arise when advanced procedures are practiced in live patients. This article discusses the Veterinary Applied Laparoscopic Training program, which provides simulation-based training for MIS.

The practice of veterinary laparoscopic surgery has grown in the past decade. Surgical devices routinely used in human laparoscopy have become available to the veterinary surgeon, at a cost the veterinary market can bear. This includes electrosurgical generators, access ports, stapling devices, tissue dissectors, and a wide array of laparoscopic handpieces. With the development of the laparoscopic clip applier in the 1990s, laparoscopic cholecystectomy came to be commonly performed in people. During this time, numerous training programs were developed to rapidly bring human surgeons up to speed.

Anesthesia for endoscopic surgery can be challenging depending on surgical manipulations and patient comorbidity. Anesthetists must understand the possible systemic changes and complications that are associated with endoscopic surgery. Pneumoperitoneum induces vasoconstriction, reduces cardiac output, and decreases functional residual capacity in the cardiopulmonary system. Both hypoventilation caused by the thoracoscopic procedure and CO_2 insufflation increase $Paco_2$. To prevent the problems associated with high $Paco_2$, monitoring of end-tidal CO_2 ($ETco_2$) and capability of positive pressure ventilation are crucial. Sudden changes of $ETco_2$ should be monitored closely. Endoscopic surgery should be a less invasive procedure; however, appropriate analgesia remains necessary.

Laparoscopic-assisted procedures allow a balance between the improved patient recoveries often associated with smaller incisions and the need for appropriate visualization of visceral organs and identification of lesions. The organ systems of small animal veterinary patients that are highly amenable to laparoscopic-assisted procedures include the urinary bladder, the gastrointestinal tract, and the reproductive tracts. Laparoscopic-assisted procedures are especially beneficial in the approach to luminal organs, allowing the organ incision to be exteriorized through the body wall, protecting the peritoneal cavity from contamination from luminal contents. Procedure-specific morbidities and patient selection should be considered when choosing between assisted laparoscopic and open approaches.

Recently, a new platform of abdominal access, called single-port surgery, has emerged in human and veterinary laparoscopy. The single-port platform enables all laparoscopic instruments, including the telescope, to pass individually through the same abdominal incision. Recently, there have been several published reports documenting the efficacy and safety of single-port procedures in veterinary patients. This article discusses the common single-port devices and instrumentation, as well as procedures now routinely offered in veterinary minimally invasive surgery.

Flexible endoscopy, a minimally invasive diagnostic and potentially therapeutic tool, has become more available over the past decades. A fiberscope is used to visualize the lumen of the area of interest and collect tissue or fluid samples for evaluation. Samples can be submitted for histopathology, cytologic analysis, and bacterial culture. Flexible endoscopy is being investigated. This article provides a brief review of equipment and basic flexible endoscopy followed by an overview of advanced flexible endoscopic procedures that focuses on the gastrointestinal tract. The procedures included here may become more readily available and improve diagnosis and treatment.

The use of endoscopy in veterinary medicine has become the mainstay of diagnosis and treatment in the subspecialty of small animal urology over the past decade. This subspecialty is termed endourology. With the common incidence of urinary tract obstructions, stones disease, renal disease, and urothelial malignancies, combined with the recognized invasiveness and morbidity associated with traditional surgical techniques, the use of endoscopic-assisted alternatives using interventional endoscopic techniques has become appealing to both owners and clinicians. This article

provides a brief overview of some of the most common urologic procedures being performed in veterinary medicine.

MaryAnn G. Radlinsky

Endoscopic surgery is a rapidly expanding modality of diagnosis and treatment of small animal patients. The development of skills, equipment, and
minimally invasive means of correcting complications may be of great
importance in decreasing the incidence of conversion from endoscopic
to open surgery; however, conversion to an open approach should never
be seen as a failure. Conversion should be considered at any time it is of
the greatest benefit for the patient. This concept is important enough to
warrant discussion with the owner before surgery and acceptance of the
need to convert without further consultation during the procedure.

Joseph Brad Case

Video-assisted thoracic surgery (VATS) is an evolving modality in the treatment and management of a variety of pathologies affecting dogs and cats.
Representative disease processes include pericardial effusion, pericardial
neoplasia, cranial mediastinal neoplasia, vascular ring anomaly, pulmonary neoplasia, pulmonary blebs and bullae, spontaneous pneumothorax,
and chylothorax. Several descriptive and small case reports have been
published on the use of VATS in veterinary medicine. More recently, larger
case series and experimental studies have revealed potential benefits and
limitations not documented previously. Significant technological advances
over the past 5 years have made possible a host of new applications in
VATS. This article focuses on updates and cutting-edge applications in
VATS.

MaryAnn G. Radlinsky

Ear disease is a common condition in dogs and cats, and otoscopy should
be performed on every case. Video-otoscopy is an incredible tool for the
diagnosis, treatment, and management of ear disease. It may serve as a
form of positive reinforcement because the client can readily see progress
made with treatment. This article focuses on the proper use of video-
otoscopy for the diagnosis, treatment, and management of ear diseases
in dogs and cats. Proper anatomy, equipment, and diagnostic understanding are required to minimize the risk of recurrent or chronic otitis, which is a
source of discomfort for the patient and frustration for the owner and the
clinician.

VETERINARY CLINICS OF NORTH AMERICA: SMALL ANIMAL PRACTICE

RELATED INTEREST

Veterinary Clinics of North America: Exotic Animal Practice
September 2015, Volume 18, Issue 3
Endoscopy
Stephen J. Divers and Laila M. Proença, *Editors*

THE CLINICS ARE NOW AVAILABLE ONLINE!
Access your subscription at:
www.theclinics.com

Preface
Endoscopy

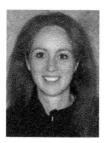

MaryAnn G. Radlinsky, DVM, MS
Editor

This issue of *Veterinary Clinics of North America*: *Small Animal Practice* focuses on minimally invasive surgery (MIS). MIS is an ever-expanding field in veterinary medicine and surgery. We have definitely gone beyond diagnostic endoscopy and greatly developed our range of therapeutic procedures. It seems that we are not only discovering the utility of procedures currently done in people, but we are also expanding MIS in veterinary patients through the creativity of people like the authors in this issue. Becoming more aggressive in types of procedures requires, and has benefited from, advances in technology, and veterinarians have been exposed to the new technology in a relatively rapid fashion. Performing more challenging procedures also requires vigilant patient care and monitoring during and after MIS. Our colleagues in anesthesia have kindly supported and tolerated our endeavors! A multidisciplinary approach is extremely helpful and appreciated. This issue has also examined advances in laparoscopic, flexible endoscopic, thoracoscopic, and urinary tract procedures. The future is certainly rife with soon to be discovered advances that will surpass those of this issue, and we welcome the hard work of clinicians that challenge themselves, and us, to do more with MIS. With advancement comes side effects, complications, and conditions of which to be aware, and for which we must monitor. Finally, MIS is becoming more prevalent in veterinary surgery, and advancement of training and maintaining skills in the field will be part of the future in training veterinary surgeons and others interested in this ever-expanding field.

I send a hearty THANK YOU to the contributing authors for this issue. Your work on these articles, and in the advancement of MIS in veterinary medicine and surgery, is

Vet Clin Small Anim 46 (2016) ix–x
http://dx.doi.org/10.1016/j.cvsm.2015.10.001
0195-5616/16/$ – see front matter © 2016 Published by Elsevier Inc.

vetsmall.theclinics.com

greatly appreciated. It is hoped that this issue is a resource, and source, of inspiration for current and future veterinarians, and for further development in the field.

MaryAnn G. Radlinsky, DVM, MS
Department of Small Animal
Medicine & Surgery
College of Veterinary Medicine
The University of Georgia
501 D.W. Brooks Drive
Athens, GA, USA

E-mail address:
makorad@gmail.com

Advances in Laparoscopic Skills Training and Management

Boel A. Fransson, DVM, PhD

KEYWORDS

- Simulation • Minimally invasive surgery • VALT • Training

KEY POINTS

- Effective laparoscopic skills training programs are not available for veterinary practitioners, but such training opportunity is required for patient safety reasons if veterinary minimally invasive surgery (MIS) is to expand.
- Basic laparoscopic skills are best trained in simulators for ethical, cost, and efficiency reasons.
- The veterinary assessment of laparoscopic skills (VALS) laparoscopic simulation training program is designed for veterinarians and will be offered at several institutions nationally and internationally.
- Ten hours of practice is required for minimum basic skills competency, but mastery requires 10,000 hours of deliberate practice.
- Simulation training is only a part of laparoscopic skills training; cadaver or high-fidelity model work is also necessary if the learning curve is to be moved out of the operating room.

LAPAROSCOPIC SKILLS TRAINING

Veterinarians interested in adding MIS to their surgical repertoire will discover the need for a distinct set of skills. The use of long instruments magnifies tremor and limits tactile sensation, often referred to as haptic feedback. The instrument portal limits instrument movement and results in a fulcrum effect, and the surgeon loses freedom to simply alter the approaching angle. In addition, depth perception is lost as normal binocular vision becomes monocular via the camera. The field of view is restricted compared with the bird's eye view of the entire body cavity associated with open surgery, and any instrument activity outside the view becomes a liability.

The author has no financial disclosures. Washington State University is a VALS test center and when launched will offer the VALS program as a cost-to-cover operation.
Department of Veterinary Clinical Sciences, Washington State University, 100 Ott Way, Pullman, WA 99164-6610, USA
E-mail address: bfransso@vetmed.wsu.edu

These MIS skills do not transfer from open surgery; they require specific training. Training by the conventional paradigm of "see-one-do-one-teach-one" is not adequate for MIS. Training based solely on practice in live patients becomes limited and inconsistent. In addition, ethical and cost issues arise when advanced procedures are practiced in live patients. Despite these challenges, the veterinary profession has been able to produce several competent and highly skilled minimally invasive surgeons. These individuals have in common a passion for pioneering veterinary MIS. The challenge for the future consists in training of a larger number of surgeons to expand the breadth and application of veterinary MIS. Even experienced veterinary laparoscopic surgeons tend to lag in efficient use of their nondominant hand, something easily rectified by simulation training.[1]

It has been stated that basic laparoscopic skills are most efficiently trained through simulation training[2]; this has been recognized for more than a decade among medical doctors (MDs), and since 2008, laparoscopic simulation training curricula have been a requirement for MD surgery residency programs in the United States.[3] Robust evidence has been presented to demonstrate that skills developed by simulation indeed transfers into improved operating room performance.[4–6] Recent systematic review has shown that simulation training of MD surgeons benefits patients by faster surgery times and higher likelihood of same-day discharge.[7]

SIMULATION MODELS

Simulation training is excellent for practicing basic laparoscopic skills. Several specific psychomotor skills have been identified as being required in MIS: ambidexterity, hand-eye coordination, instrument targeting accuracy, and recognition of depth cues.[8,9] These skills can be trained effectively in a variety of simulation models.

Box trainers (video trainers) use traditional laparoscopic instruments (**Fig. 1**) and an inexpensive Web camera placed within the box, which projects the real-time image on a television or computer screen. In contrast, virtual reality (VR) training entails a variety of computer-generated exercises and surgical procedures, also exposing the trainee to simulated complications such as bleeding, iatrogenic trauma to the peritoneal lining, and bile leakage. A hybrid type of trainer, augmented reality trainer combines the traditional box trainer with a VR environment. At present, there is no conclusive evidence to indicate that one type of training model is superior to another.[10–13] A summary of the main advantages and disadvantages with these different training models are presented in (**Table 1**).

SETTING UP A TRAINING PROGRAM

Simulation training facilities are limited for veterinarians. Likewise, few laparoscopic training programs have been designed for veterinary surgeons. The author's institution has trained residents and surgeons since 2008, in the Veterinary Applied Laparoscopic Training (VALT) laboratory (see **Fig. 1**). The author has also researched training methods (residents, surgeons, and novices).[1,14,15] The initial VALT training programs used box trainers and physical models.[1] At present, data from a study comparing training programs using multimodal training, including VR, box training, and physical models, are being analyzed. Preliminary results indicate that the type of exercises does not lead to major differences in outcome. Similar observations have also been made at other centers.[16] There is, however, no doubt that simulation training of some form is necessary, and both box training and VR training have robust evidence linking them to improved operating performance, shortening surgery times and decreasing hospitalization length.[7,17]

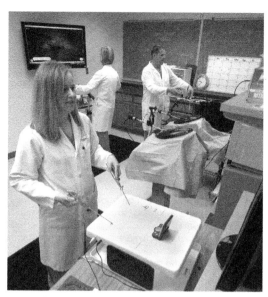

Fig. 1. The Veterinary Applied Laparoscopic Training (VALT) laboratory at Washington State University uses several types of simulation trainers. Clockwise from top left in the image a virtual reality trainer projected on a wall-mounted flat-screen television (TV), canine abdominal models used with standard laparoscopic instrumentation, and a box trainer (video trainer) using low-fidelity simulation with a Web camera image projected real time on a TV screen. (*Courtesy of* Henry Moore, College of Veterinary Medicine, Washington State University, Pullman, WA.)

Several important lessons have been learnt through the work in the VALT laboratory in how to design training programs. The importance of deliberate practice cannot be overstated; expert performance results from deliberately engaging in and choosing specific training tasks that improve and maintain high performance.[18] Such training requires repeated practice and appropriate feedback, which allow the trainee to focus on weaknesses and refine performance.[18] Training without clear goals and feedback lead to an early plateau in the trainees' skills,[19] although being as expensive and time consuming as an effective program. The principles of deliberate practice (**Box 1**) outlines that an effective training program consists of (1) tasks with well-defined goals, (2) trainees who are motivated to improve, and (3) trainees who are provided individual and targeted feedback, and (4) trainees who are given ample opportunity for repetition and refinement. This concept explains why simply buying expensive equipment for simulation training without providing the trainee with selected training tasks, dedicated time for training, and individual instruction and feedback is likely to fail.

Training Tasks

Training of the basic skills of ambidexterity, hand-eye coordination, instrument targeting accuracy, and recognition of depth cues has been proved effective by both box training and VR training.[11,20] However, the advanced skills of suturing and knot tying have traditionally been considered better trained in physical models (box training), which provide haptic feedback, rather than in VR.[21] A new generation of VR trainers with haptic feedback is available, but the benefits are still debated.[20,22,23] Training in VR carries several different advantages, as the tasks are well defined and instructions and feedback are built into the software. For box training, there are many

Table 1
Advantages and disadvantages of different simulation models

Simulation Type	Advantages	Disadvantages
Box trainers	• Low cost; commercial systems are inexpensive, and homemade versions can also be used • Haptic feedback • Versatile • Validated training goals and programs[1,24] are available	• Requires expert observer for feedback and instruction • Requires disposable training materials such as suture, ligature loops, and cutting material
Virtual reality trainers	• High-fidelity simulations, including complete surgical procedures • Enables practice of complication management (bleeding, soft-tissue trauma) • Simulates use of expensive equipment, electrocautery, clip application, and so on • No need for disposable materials • Automated feedback, with comparison to experts • Provide metrics measurements such as time, instrument movement, and errors	• High cost • Haptic feedback either lacking or not consistently realistic[22] • No veterinary models available; human anatomy simulated • The expert performance values are not standardized[25,26]
Augmented reality trainers	Combines haptic feedback from box training with virtual reality trainer advantages	Limited availability[40]
Higher-fidelity physical models for veterinarians	• Simulated canine abdomen (Sawbones, Vashon, WA, USA) gives realistic confines of the canine abdomen • Future higher-fidelity models may provide opportunity for veterinary surgical procedure training in box trainers	Limited availability

validated and well-described tasks available. Dr Rosser at Yale University developed a series of station tasks in the 1990s used in the popular "Top-Gun Shoot-Out" competition consisting of a cobra rope drill, pea drop drill, terrible triangle drill, and suturing drill. However, the most solidly validated tasks are those described by Dr Fried's group at McGill University, Canada.[2] These tasks have been described under the acronym of MISTELS, the McGill inanimate simulator for training and evaluation of laparoscopic skills, and are now incorporated in the high-stakes test of MD surgeons, the Fundamentals of Laparoscopic Surgery (FLS). Subsequently, the MISTELS tasks have served as the foundation for the first training/assessment program developed for veterinary use, the VALS program (**Fig. 2**), which is in the final development stages to be launched late 2015. The following tasks are incorporated in the VALS program:

1. Pegboard transfer: Laparoscopic grasping forceps in the nondominant hand is used to lift each of 6 pegs from a pegboard, transfer them to a grasper in the dominant hand, place them on a second pegboard, and finally reverse the exercise (**Fig. 3**).

> **Box 1**
> **Training programs based on these principles of deliberate practice maximizes the benefits of training**
>
> 1. Tasks with well-defined goals
> 2. Trainee's motivation to improve
> 3. Trainee provided with feedback
> 4. Ample opportunity for repetition and gradual refinement of performance
>
> *Modified from* Ericsson KA. Deliberate practice and the acquisition and maintenance of expert performance in medicine and related domains. Acad Med 2004;79:S70–81.

2. Pattern cutting: This task involves cutting a 4-cm-diameter circular pattern out of a 10 × 15-cm piece of instrument wrapping material or a gauze, suspended between alligator clips (**Fig. 4**).
3. Ligature loop placement: The task involves placing a ligature loop pre-tied with a laparoscopic slip knot over a mark placed on a foam appendix and cinch it down with a disposable-type knot pusher (**Fig. 5**).
4. Extracorporeal suturing: A simple interrupted suture using long (90-cm) suture on a taper-point needle is placed through marked needle entry and exit points in a slit Penrose drain segment. The first throw in the knot is tied extracorporeally with a slip knot and cinched down by use of a knot pusher. Thereafter, 3 single square throws are placed by use of laparoscopic needle holders and the suture is cut (**Fig. 6**).
5. Intracorporeal suturing: A simple interrupted suture is placed using short (12- to 15-cm-long) suture on a taper-point needle through marked needle entry and exit points in a slit Penrose drain segment. Three throws are placed, the first being a surgeon's (double) throw, by use of laparoscopic needle holders. The exercise is completed when the suture is cut (**Fig. 7**).

The selected training tasks need to be demonstrated to the trainee, usually by depicting the correct performance in narrated video tutorials. In addition, the performance goals need to be clearly stated, which makes use of validated tasks with likewise validated goals such as MISTELS and VALS advantageous.[24] In VR training, the performance goals are the expert performance level provided in the software. However, some of these performance goals, including motion metrics, have been criticized for inconsistency[25–27] and may need to be refined.

After achieving basic skills and suturing competency through simulation training, the trainee needs access to surgical procedure task training in high-fidelity models,

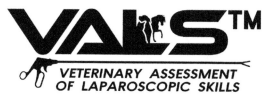

Fig. 2. The logotype for the upcoming VALS program, aiming to make simulation training accessible nationally and internationally to veterinary practitioners. The VALS program will combine training modules with certification of skills, basic (PreVALS) and advanced (VALS). (*Courtesy of* VALS-TM, with permission from Washington State University, 2015, Pullman, WA.)

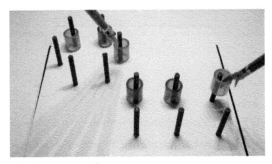

Fig. 3. The first VALS task, peg transfer.

cadaver, and/or live animal models. Simulation training is not yet available for the important tasks of establishing instrument portals and creating a pneumoperitoneum for working space. These tasks are imperative for surgical success and need to be mastered by a veterinary surgeon. To some extent, cannula placement and insufflation can be trained in the operating room because the performance is fairly standardized, but these surgical tasks are also among the most risk-filled parts of MIS.[28] For ethical reasons, cannula placement should ideally be trained in inanimate models or in cadaver models. VR trainers offer surgical procedure training but cannot replace animal work, as all available VR is programmed for human anatomy and physiology. In addition, VR models mainly focus on instrument handling, not on portal placement. Future work on training programs might outline that the ideal surgeon's training starts with simulation training and then progresses via cadaver or high-fidelity model work to live animal work.

Motivation of Trainees

A major limitation when training veterinary surgeons and residents is to ensure motivation to training, in the face of long working hours and a high load of clinical responsibilities. This trainee group is in general highly motivated to enhance skills, but a training program that relies on internal motivation among the trainees as the sole motivator is doomed to failure. Even when technologically advanced training equipment is made available to residents, voluntary participation is limited to between 6% and 14%.[29,30] External motivation, such as mandating training and punitive measures if not attending training, has shown to be an effective strategy.[27] A recent survey among MD residents indicate that a mandatory simulation training program, with protected time, is a prerequisite for participation.[31] This perception is supported by studies

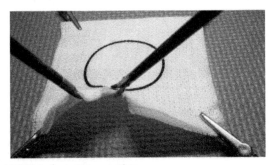

Fig. 4. The second VALS task, pattern cutting.

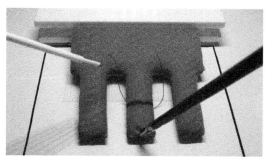

Fig. 5. The third VALS task, ligature loop placement.

demonstrating that dedicated regular time for training, known ahead of time to trainees and their faculty mentors, led to increased participation.[29,30] In the VALT laboratory, there have been challenges with motivation, especially among surgeons. Not unexpectedly, the MIS experience level of the participant was inversely related to the motivation to practice.[1] This important finding illuminates that simulation training preferably starts early in the career of the MIS surgeon, ideally before or simultaneously with the first exposure to MIS in the operating room. The VALT laboratory has worked with mandatory training sessions but on a flexible time schedule, to which the trainees sign up on a Web-based schedule. Resident trainees also tend to be graduate students, and the combination of graduate studies and clinical residency training has not allowed us to dedicate a specific hour for practice. Equipment limitations have also made it advantageous to spread out training sessions. A key point worth highlighting is the role of a dedicated laboratory manager who ensures training completion and can remind participants who lag behind. Furthermore, clearly demonstrated commitment of the faculty, by supporting the training and taking an active role in instruction, makes trainees highly motivated.

Fortunately for the educator, the target group for MIS training tends to be highly competitive personalities. Most training tasks are based on metrics including time for completion, which is an easy goal to measure. Setting appropriate training goals entails a strong internal motivation. Even better, scheduled assessments with scoring of performance serves to greatly enhance internal motivation. The upcoming VALS program offers certification for 2 skills tests: a basic test, the Preliminary-VALS (PreVALS) test, and the actual VALS test including the advanced suturing and knot-tying skills. Availability of a standardized certifiable skills test will likely serve as a strong motivator for simulation training.

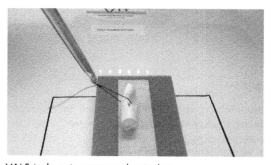

Fig. 6. The fourth VALS task, extracorporeal suturing.

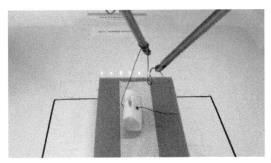

Fig. 7. The fifth VALS task, intracorporeal suturing.

Feedback

One of the most important principles for deliberate practice is individual and targeted feedback. Training in VR is appealing as motion metrics are built into the software, and such feedback is valuable. However, the most powerful feedback is verbal, individual, detailed, and provided by an expert observing the trainee's performance.[32] In the ideal training program, the trainee receives individualized feedback, and subsequent training tailored to such feedback has been demonstrated to greatly improve operating room performance.[33] Feedback, if perceived by the trainee as relevant, serves both as a guide and a powerful motivator for further training.

Ample Opportunity to Practice

As previously stated, the training opportunities for aspiring veterinary MIS surgeons are severely limited. However, a movement to make VALS simulation training available to veterinary residents and practitioners is gaining momentum. It is hoped that such training and certification will be available to most surgery residents within a couple of years. Training for MD surgeons followed a similar trajectory approximately a decade ago. In 2006, roughly half of residency programs had simulation training programs, whereas by 2008, such training laboratories became mandatory for all residency training programs.[3] The VALT laboratory at the authors' institution offers veterinarians training, but for deliberate practice of skills and skills retention, trainees need opportunity for sustained training. Short-course-type training leads to inferior skills acquisition when compared with distributed practice.[27] Although not entirely understood, it seems as if the optimal training program consists of 1-hour sessions, at most once daily,[34] with a rest period in between allowing for cerebral internalization of the learning. Approximately 10 hours of training has shown sufficient for passing of the FLS test, that is, demonstrating basic manual skills competency.[24] However, for the surgeon aspiring for expert performance and mastery, the requirement is probably closer to 10,000 hours of deliberate practice.[18,35]

SURGEON SELF-TRAINING

Most practicing veterinarians will not have access to sustained organized skills training programs within the foreseeable future. However, basic laparoscopic psychomotor skills can be achieved by independent practice of MISTELS/VALS-type of exercises as outlined earlier. The tasks in those programs are well defined, and the goals are easy to monitor. The FLS self-study guidelines state that if the participant consistently can perform a 53-second peg transfer, 50-second pattern cut, 87-second ligature loop, 99-second extracorporeal suturing, and 96-second intracorporeal suturing times, the vast majority can pass the FLS test.[36] Corresponding performance goals for VALS are likely to be available in the future, and owing to the similarities of the tests, these performance goals may not be vastly different. For the surgeon with limited funding available for purchase of training material, there are affordable alternatives to the VALS training box available, such as those from the United Kingdom–based company eoSurgical (Bergamo, UK). In addition, the quality of Web cameras today is such that one can easily construct homemade versions of box trainers and use a laptop for real-time projection (**Figs. 8** and **9**).

The dedicated aspiring MIS surgeon could thus achieve basic skills by simulation training and thereafter complement with live-model short-course training, which is often offered in cooperation with industry such as Karl Storz (for courses see http://www.karlstorzvet.com/education.html). Before implementing MIS in clinical practice, cadaver training for cannula placement and pneumoperitoneum insufflation is advisable. After consulting current textbooks regarding the surgical technique, the surgeon is thereafter likely able to start with entry-level surgical procedures, including laparoscopic ovariectomy, ovariohysterectomy, and several laparoscopy-assisted techniques.

VIDEO GAMES

There is mounting evidence that video games may provide a useful addition to laparoscopic skills training. A systematic review has concluded that novices and laparoscopic surgeons with ongoing video game experience have superior laparoscopic simulator skills.[37] Meta-analysis has pointed out that video gaming seems to lead to higher baseline laparoscopic skills score and effective warming up before laparoscopic surgery.[38] However, standardized methods to assess video game experience are needed for future work.[38] Millard and colleagues[39] have pioneered work on video gaming and laparoscopic skills in veterinary medicine. A positive correlation between video game proficiency and laparoscopic box-trainer proficiency was noted. It was concluded that video games may represent an underutilized training modality, which in the future could serve as an inexpensive and effective adjunct to simulation training of laparoscopic skills.

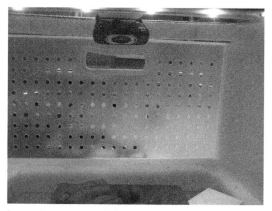

Fig. 8. Homemade box trainers can easily be made by use of a high–frame rate Web camera.

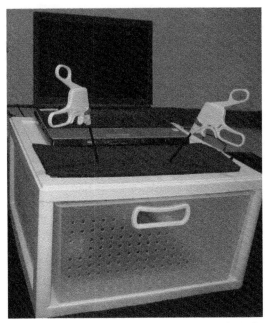

Fig. 9. An example of a homemade box trainer used in the author's laparoscopic training laboratory.

MAINTAINING SKILLS

Superior skills retention is the main argument for sustained distributed laparoscopic skills training, as compared with short-course, massed training.[34] Trainees who have achieved proficiency goals in distributed training have been shown to retain those skills up to 5 to 6 months.[5,34] Therefore, laparoscopic simulation training should be revisited approximately biannually for surgeons and residents who have achieved basic skills competency. In the author's opinion, the advantages of having continuous access to a laparoscopic simulation laboratory are numerous. The skills laboratory allows for continuous training of residents, for refreshing every 6 months for surgeons, and for warm-up practice in preparation for advanced cases. It is hoped that veterinary medicine will parallel the development of the MDs and see an increasing number of skills laboratories developing during the next decade, to where simulation training is readily accessible for all veterinary surgeons. Ultimately, patients would benefit by decreased morbidity and increased surgeon confidence.

REFERENCES

1. Fransson BA, Ragle CA, Bryan ME. Effects of two training curricula on basic laparoscopic skills and surgical performance among veterinarians. J Am Vet Med Assoc 2012;241:451–60.
2. Fried GM, Feldman LS, Vassiliou MC, et al. Proving the value of simulation in laparoscopic surgery. Ann Surg 2004;240:518–25 [discussion: 525–8].
3. Scott DJ, Dunnington GL. The new ACS/APDS skills curriculum: moving the learning curve out of the operating room. J Gastrointest Surg 2008;12:213–21.

4. Korndorffer JR Jr, Dunne JB, Sierra R, et al. Simulator training for laparoscopic suturing using performance goals translates to the operating room. J Am Coll Surg 2005;201:23–9.
5. Stefanidis D, Acker C, Heniford BT. Proficiency-based laparoscopic simulator training leads to improved operating room skill that is resistant to decay. Surg Innov 2008;15:69–73.
6. Dawe SR, Pena GN, Windsor JA, et al. Systematic review of skills transfer after surgical simulation-based training. Br J Surg 2014;101:1063–76.
7. Gurusamy KS, Nagendran M, Toon CD, et al. Laparoscopic surgical box model training for surgical trainees with limited prior laparoscopic experience. Cochrane Database Syst Rev 2014;(3):CD010478.
8. Derossis AM, Fried GM, Abrahamowicz M, et al. Development of a model for training and evaluation of laparoscopic skills. Am J Surg 1998;175:482–7.
9. Rosser JC Jr, Rosser LE, Savalgi RS. Objective evaluation of a laparoscopic surgical skill program for residents and senior surgeons. Arch Surg 1998;133:657–61.
10. Debes AJ, Aggarwal R, Balasundaram I, et al. A tale of two trainers: virtual reality versus a video trainer for acquisition of basic laparoscopic skills. Am J Surg 2010;199:840–5.
11. Diesen DL, Erhunmwunsee L, Bennett KM, et al. Effectiveness of laparoscopic computer simulator versus usage of box trainer for endoscopic surgery training of novices. J Surg Educ 2011;68:282–9.
12. Jensen K, Ringsted C, Hansen HJ, et al. Simulation-based training for thoracoscopic lobectomy: a randomized controlled trial: virtual-reality versus black-box simulation. Surg Endosc 2014;28:1821–9.
13. Mohammadi Y, Lerner MA, Sethi AS, et al. Comparison of laparoscopy training using the box trainer versus the virtual trainer. JSLS 2010;14:205–12.
14. Fransson BA, Ragle CA. Assessment of laparoscopic skills before and after simulation training with a canine abdominal model. J Am Vet Med Assoc 2010;236:1079–84.
15. Fransson BA, Ragle CA, Bryan ME. A laparoscopic surgical skills assessment tool for veterinarians. J Vet Med Educ 2010;37:304–13.
16. Brinkman WM, Havermans SY, Buzink SN, et al. Single versus multimodality training basic laparoscopic skills. Surg Endosc 2012;26:2172–8.
17. Nagendran M, Gurusamy KS, Aggarwal R, et al. Virtual reality training for surgical trainees in laparoscopic surgery. Cochrane Database Syst Rev 2013;(8):CD006575.
18. Ericsson KA. Deliberate practice and the acquisition and maintenance of expert performance in medicine and related domains. Acad Med 2004;79:S70–81.
19. Hashimoto DA, Sirimanna P, Gomez ED, et al. Deliberate practice enhances quality of laparoscopic surgical performance in a randomized controlled trial: from arrested development to expert performance. Surg Endosc 2014. [Epub ahead of print].
20. Beyer-Berjot L, Aggarwal R. Toward technology-supported surgical training: the potential of virtual simulators in laparoscopic surgery. Scand J Surg 2013;102:221–6.
21. Botden SM, Torab F, Buzink SN, et al. The importance of haptic feedback in laparoscopic suturing training and the additive value of virtual reality simulation. Surg Endosc 2008;22:1214–22.
22. Vapenstad C, Hofstad EF, Lango T, et al. Perceiving haptic feedback in virtual reality simulators. Surg Endosc 2013;27:2391–7.

23. Willis RE, Gomez PP, Ivatury SJ, et al. Virtual reality simulators: valuable surgical skills trainers or video games? J Surg Educ 2014;71:426–33.

24. Scott DJ, Ritter EM, Tesfay ST, et al. Certification pass rate of 100% for fundamentals of laparoscopic surgery skills after proficiency-based training. Surg Endosc 2008;22:1887–93.

25. Thijssen AS, Schijven MP. Contemporary virtual reality laparoscopy simulators: quicksand or solid grounds for assessing surgical trainees? Am J Surg 2010; 199:529–41.

26. Luursema JM, Rovers MM, Alken A, et al. When experts are oceans apart: comparing expert performance values for proficiency-based laparoscopic simulator training. J Surg Educ 2015;72(3):536–41.

27. Stefanidis D, Heniford BT. The formula for a successful laparoscopic skills curriculum. Arch Surg 2009;144:77–82 [discussion: 82].

28. Compeau C, McLeod NT, Ternamian A. Laparoscopic entry: a review of Canadian general surgical practice. Can J Surg 2011;54:315–20.

29. Stefanidis D, Acker CE, Swiderski D, et al. Challenges during the implementation of a laparoscopic skills curriculum in a busy general surgery residency program. J Surg Educ 2008;65:4–7.

30. Chang L, Petros J, Hess DT, et al. Integrating simulation into a surgical residency program: is voluntary participation effective? Surg Endosc 2007;21:418–21.

31. Shetty S, Zevin B, Grantcharov TP, et al. Perceptions, training experiences, and preferences of surgical residents toward laparoscopic simulation training: a resident survey. J Surg Educ 2014;71:727–33.

32. Porte MC, Xeroulis G, Reznick RK, et al. Verbal feedback from an expert is more effective than self-accessed feedback about motion efficiency in learning new surgical skills. Am J Surg 2007;193:105–10.

33. Palter VN, Grantcharov TP. Individualized deliberate practice on a virtual reality simulator improves technical performance of surgical novices in the operating room: a randomized controlled trial. Ann Surg 2014;259:443–8.

34. De Win G, Van Bruwaene S, De Ridder D, et al. The optimal frequency of endoscopic skill labs for training and skill retention on suturing: a randomized controlled trial. J Surg Educ 2013;70:384–93.

35. Ericsson KA, Prietula MJ, Cokely ET. The making of an expert. Harv Bus Rev 2007;85:114–21, 193.

36. Cassera MA, Zheng B, Swanstrom LL. Data-based self-study guidelines for the fundamentals of laparoscopic surgery examination. Surg Endosc 2012;26: 3426–9.

37. Ou Y, McGlone ER, Camm CF, et al. Does playing video games improve laparoscopic skills? Int J Surg 2013;11:365–9.

38. Jalink MB, Goris J, Heineman E, et al. The effects of video games on laparoscopic simulator skills. Am J Surg 2014;208:151–6.

39. Millard HA, Millard RP, Constable PD, et al. Relationships among video gaming proficiency and spatial orientation, laparoscopic, and traditional surgical skills of third-year veterinary students. J Am Vet Med Assoc 2014;244:357–62.

40. Botden SM, Jakimowicz JJ. What is going on in augmented reality simulation in laparoscopic surgery? Surg Endosc 2009;23:1693–700.

Advances in Equipment and Instrumentation in Laparoscopic Surgery

John C. Huhn, DVM, MS

KEYWORDS

- Laparoscopy • Equipment • Instruments • Electrosurgery • Stapling • Endoscopy
- Suturing

KEY POINTS

- Several methods of laparoscopic access (Veress needle, Hasson method, Single incision laparoscopic surgery, threaded and optical ports) are available.
- The laparoscopic access method is of primary importance in determining instrument options (articulating or straight) and manipulative methods (direct or indirect triangulation).
- Laparoscopic suturing equipment (assisted suturing devices, endoscopic needle holders, barbed sutures) and familiarity with its use provide greater versatility to the laparoscopic surgeon.
- Hemorrhage control is a central principle in laparoscopic surgery, and several options (electrosurgical and endomechanical) exist to address this issue.
- Endoscopic staplers may be indicated when solid organ hemostasis is needed in thick tissue applications.

In 2005, a study was conducted to evaluate postoperative pain in female dogs sterilized laparoscopically compared with those altered via a conventional, open approach.[1] Prior to that time, sporadic reports of laparoscopic ovariohysterectomy existed in the literature, but none that specifically evaluated postoperative pain. The 2005 study demonstrated that patients undergoing laparoscopic spay exhibited significantly less pain than their open surgery counterparts.[1] This seminal study opened the door for laparoscopic ovariohysterectomy (LOH) and ovariectomy (LOE) to become the most widely practiced veterinary laparoscopic procedure. At present, nearly every veterinary laparoscopic training course teaches LOH or LOE to its participants. Not only is this surgery clinically relevant, but it presents an excellent opportunity for psychomotor skill enhancement.

Dr J.C. Huhn is a paid employee of Medtronic plc, formerly Covidien LLC.
Animal Health, Medtronic, 15 Forsyth Road, Salem, CT 06420, USA
E-mail address: John.Huhn@Covidien.com

Vet Clin Small Anim 46 (2016) 13–29
http://dx.doi.org/10.1016/j.cvsm.2015.08.005
0195-5616/16/$ – see front matter © 2016 Elsevier Inc. All rights reserved.

vetsmall.theclinics.com

LAPAROSCOPIC ACCESS

Effective laparoscopic access is critical to the success of any laparoscopic procedure. The rigid telescope, retraction devices, and operative instruments must all be appropriately positioned to provide access to the target tissue.

Threaded Metal Port

A threaded metal cannula with reducing seals has been available for some time. The fact that this device is reusable and steam autoclavable makes it appealing to veterinary surgeons. It is designed to allow insertion of a 0° rigid telescope down its shaft during insertion into the abdomen via a twisting motion. A recent design improvement features a stopper, which maintains the telescope in optimal position during cannula advancement. The spiraling ridges of the cannula terminate in a protrusion at the cannula tip. Surgeons need to be cautious during advancement through the body wall and into the abdomen, as iatrogenic damage is possible if adequate visualization is not maintained.

Optical Port

An inherent difficulty in placing laparoscopic ports lies in their atraumatic placement. This is particularly true when placing the first port, which is usually for the rigid telescope. Use of a Veress needle to insufflate the abdomen prior to port placement has been described extensively.[1-5] It is a safe and reliable method and saves significant operative time. Once the abdomen has been inflated, an optical port can be inserted under direct visualization into the abdomen. The first such devices contained an integrated cutting blade, which became dull after a single use. An improved design that does not feature a cutting blade has since been developed (**Fig. 1**). The new optical port has a ribbed, translucent cannula and a conical dolphin tip. This device is inserted into the abdomen with a twisting motion, allowing visualization of the separating muscle and fascial layers until peritoneal penetration is achieved.

SINGLE INCISION LAPAROSCOPIC SURGERY

Laparoscopic spay procedures were initially performed as 2 or 3 port techniques.[6-8] The telescope was placed in a position on midline, caudal to the umbilicus. Instrument ports were placed either on midline or lateral to the umbilicus. In so doing, traditional principles of triangulation could be utilized. Over time, however, surgeons sought to perform ovariohysterectomy or ovariectomy through fewer incisions in keeping with the principles of minimally invasive surgery. Furthermore, surgeons came to realize

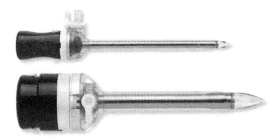

Fig. 1. Optical laparoscopic ports: 5 mm (*top*) and 5 to 12 mm (*bottom*); telescope is placed into obturator to allow visualization of abdominal entry. (*Courtesy of* Covidien, North Haven, CT; with permission. All rights reserved.)

that incisions through muscle bellies were perhaps more painful than incisions through the linea alba. As such, many surgeons came to adopt an operative method that used a more caudal midline telescope placement. Furthermore, many came to prefer an operating laparoscope, which would allow the surgeon to perform this procedure through an 11 to 12 mm incision. Therein lies the origin of the concept of single incision laparoscopic surgery, as applied to veterinary surgery.

In human surgery, single incision laparoscopic surgery (SILS) evolved from cosmetic concerns. With the position and anatomy of the human umbilicus, it became apparent that this anatomic landmark presented an optimal portal for abdominal entry. To this end, various devices were developed to allow use of the umbilicus as a laparoscopic portal. One such device is the SILS port (**Fig. 2**), whose use has been described in veterinary surgery.[9] Insertion of the SILS port (Medtronic, Minneapolis, Minnesota) requires a 2 cm incision through the abdominal wall to anchor the port. The SILS device has 4 channels, which allow insertion of 5 to 15 mm diameter cannulae. As such, 5 mm handpieces, 5 to 12 mm telescopes, and 10 to 15 mm stapling devices can all be introduced simultaneously through a 2 cm abdominal access incision. One of the SILS channels can be used for insufflation, using a specially designed plug and tubing.

Specific instrumentation is available for usage with the SILS port. These instruments are unique in regard to allowable range of motion afforded by their design. Rotational movement can be achieved along both the shaft and the tip of most instruments. Articulation is achieved via a pivoting joint at the junction of the body and the shaft of the handpiece. Furthermore, articulation may be statically maintained via a locking trigger mechanism. All of these features function together to allow laparoscopic manipulation in a nontraditional manner. These specialized instruments are intended to be used in a cross-handed manner within the abdomen. As such, instruments held in the right hand are meant to work from the surgeon's left side within the abdomen. The same applies to instruments held with the left hand. In this scenario, the instrument shafts cross one another within the SILS port. As can be imagined, a learning curve is associated with this type of manipulation.

Many veterinary surgeons prefer to use straight instruments with the SILS system. There is a greater tendency to encounter instrument interference at the handpiece controls when using straight instruments. However, this can be overcome by staggering ports and instruments with respect to their depth within the SILS port (**Fig. 3**).

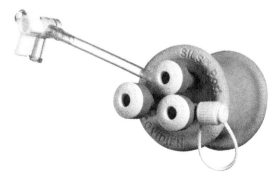

Fig. 2. SILS port: up to 4 port sites are available to accommodate the rigid telescope, surgical instruments, electrosurgical devices, and insufflation ports. A 2 cm incision is necessary to accommodate the foam donut within the abdominal wall. (*Courtesy of* Covidien; with permission. All rights reserved.)

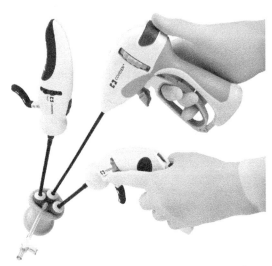

Fig. 3. Instrument and port placement in SILS port to minimize interference during telescope and instrument manipulations. (*Courtesy of* Covidien; with permission. All rights reserved.)

The reusability of the SILS port system in veterinary surgery has been investigated.[10] It was determined that the SILS foam collar could be safely sterilized to allow reuse in veterinary patients. This is an important finding, as the cost of a single-use SILS system would not be cost-effective for most veterinary surgeons.

Laparoscopic Suturing

The ability to suture laparoscopically makes a laparoscopic surgeon more versatile. Procedures that were once only possible via a laparoscopically assisted approach can now be performed via a true laparoscopic approach. Gastropexy is most notable in this regard.[11] With time, procedures such as gastrointestinal resection and anastomosis will be performed, as are routinely done in human surgery.

Barbed Sutures

Barbed sutures (**Fig. 4**) were originally developed for use in human cutaneous closure. They were meant to decrease operative time and improve cosmesis.[5] With time, genitourinary surgeons began using barbed sutures in the confined spaces of the reproductive tract.[12,13] Laparoscopic applications soon followed, given the fact that barbed sutures greatly facilitated suturing within the abdomen.

Barbed sutures are available as both bidirectional and unidirectional strands. Bidirectional barbed sutures are double-armed with suture needles and have a nonbarbed section at the midpoint of the strand. Unidirectional barbed sutures feature a suture needle at 1 end of the strand with a terminal loop at the other. Differences in barb direction and placement along the strand dictate differences in application of bidirectional versus unidirectional barbed sutures. Bidirectional barbed sutures are initially applied to allow the nonbarbed portion to reside in the center of the wound. Suturing then proceeds in opposite directions from the central portion of the wound. Unidirectional barbed sutures are usually started at the wound margin. Following the first suture bite, the end of the suture needle is passed through the terminal loop to commence closure. Both birectional and unidirectional barbed suture closures end in similar fashion.

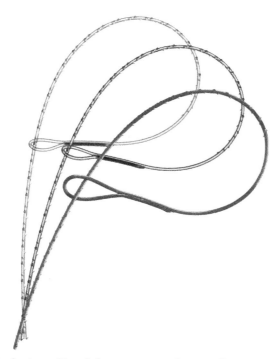

Fig. 4. VLoc barbed sutures. Strands feature a swaged-on needle at 1 end and a welded terminal loop at the other; unidirectional barbs arranged in helical configuration. Suture knotting begins with needle passage through tissue and then through terminal loop. (*Courtesy of* Covidien; with permission. All rights reserved.)

As veterinary surgeons embraced the use of barbed sutures, potential laparoscopic applications began to emerge. One such application was laparoscopic gastropexy.[14,15] The difficulty in laparoscopic gastropexy lies not only in performing intracorporeal suturing, but more specifically in tying the first suture knot, which suspends the stomach from the abdominal wall. The laparoscopist can decrease insufflation pressure, which brings the stomach and body wall into closer proximity. However, tying the first knot remains difficult without additional retraction. Unidirectional barbed sutures alleviate this problem by effectively suspending the stomach after only 2 suture passes. This greatly facilitates completion of the rest of the gastropexy. Each suture bite is maintained under local tension mediated by the helical suture barbs along the suture strand.

There is some confusion regarding suture sizing nomenclature between the major manufacturers of barbed sutures. One manufacturer designates suture size based on the outer diameter of the strand from which the barbed sutures were cut. This logically results in a suture whose central core is smaller than that of the parent strand. As such, a 3/0 suture is produced from a 2/0 parent strand, but is expected to exhibit the approximate biomechanical properties of a monofilament 3/0 strand. Another manufacturer names its barbed suture in a way that is, directly comparable to a monofilament strand of the same suture gauge. Therefore, a 3/0 barbed suture can be expected to have similar biomechanical properties to a 3/0 suture made of the same material. This apples-to-apples naming convention eliminates confusion for surgeons and operating room technicians.

AUTOMATED SUTURING DEVICES
Endo Stitch

Numerous proprietary automated suture devices have been developed in order to facilitate intracorporeal suturing. One such device is the EndoStitch (Medtronic) (**Fig. 5**), which has been available since the 1990s. The tip of the Endo Stitch features apposing jaws with holes on each side to accept a 9 mm double-taperpoint suture needle. The suture material is swaged on to the center of the needle, and is supplied in a plastic cartridge for loading into the Endo Stitch. The shaft of the device is 10 mm in diameter and is available in short (23 cm) and long (38 cm) lengths for open and laparoscopic procedures respectively. The handle portion of the Endo Stitch is controlled with 1 hand. A centrally located loading button is used to initially arm the Endo Stitch device with suture material. A swiveling toggle button located within reach of the index finger is used to transfer the suture needle from 1 jaw (armed jaw) to the other (unarmed jaw) following tissue passage and closure of the instrument tips. Suture materials available for use with the Endo Stitch include braided lactomer, silk, nylon, and polyester in 4/0 to 0 USP sizes and lengths of 7 in/18 cm to 48 in/122 cm.[16] More recently, V-LOC suture reloads have been developed for use with the Endo Stitch device (**Fig. 6**). V-LOC reloads are supplied as glycolide–trimethylene carbonate (V-LOC 180) or polybutester (V-LOC PBT) versions. V-LOC 180 reloads are absorbable and have an absorption profile similar to Maxon suture (Covidien, North Haven, CT, USA). V-LOC PBT reloads are nonabsorbable and are composed of the same material as Novafil suture (Covidien, North Haven, CT, USA). V-LOC reloads are available in sizes 3/0 to 0 and 4 in/10 cm, 6 in/15 cm, and 8 in/20 cm lengths.

Single Incision Laparoscopic Surgery Stitch

A further advance in automated suturing devices (ASDs) came with the recent introduction of the SILS Stitch (Medtronic) device (**Fig. 7**). This device represents a modification of the Endo Stitch device and is ideally suited for use with the SILS system. The SILS Stitch is essentially a roticulating Endo Stitch. It is ideally suited for use with the SILS port, as working space is limited and 2 to 3 instruments and telescope are in close proximity. The SILS Stitch has a difficult learning curve; however, suturing principles with this device are similar to those with the Endo Stitch. The challenge lies in mastering 3-dimensional manipulation while viewing a 2-dimensional operative field.

Dissecting Instruments

Laparoscopic skill development requires not only the ability to suture within the abdomen but also to perform fine dissection. To that end, specific instruments have been developed to allow tissue and vessel isolation. Nowhere is this more evident than in procedures such as adrenalectomy, cholecystectomy, and nephrectomy.

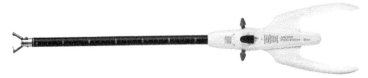

Fig. 5. Endostitch suturing device: allows one-handed intracorporeal suturing; requires the use of specialized suture loading units. (*Courtesy of* Covidien; with permission. All rights reserved.)

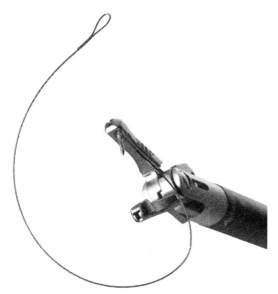

Fig. 6. Endostitch suturing device with VLoc loading unit. (*Courtesy of* Covidien; with permission. All rights reserved.)

Roticulating Maryland Dissector

It is not uncommon to place an instrument port in the abdominal wall, only to find that the angle to the target tissue is incorrect. One option is to simply place another port. However, it is often feasible to utilize an instrument such as a roticulating Maryland dissector (**Fig. 8**) to optimize the instrument approach angle. On the dissector, there

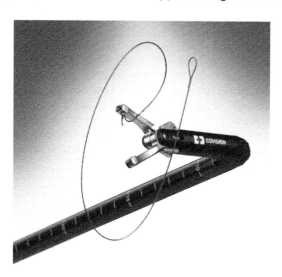

Fig. 7. SILS Stitch suturing device: functions similar to Endostitch device but with greater range of motion—rotation and articulation; much steeper learning curve. (*Courtesy of* Covidien; with permission. All rights reserved.)

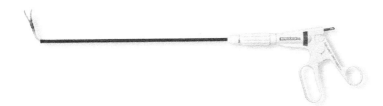

Fig. 8. Roticulating Maryland dissector. Rotational movement is achieved via green-colored wheel; movement perpendicular to the long axis of the instrument is achieved by twisting the grooved dial. (*Courtesy of* Covidien; with permission. All rights reserved.)

are controls that allow both rotation and articulation of the instrument shaft (**Fig. 9**). The instrument tip is curved and features short serrations for tissue grasping. The Maryland dissector is most useful when advanced tangentially to a vascular or tubular structure until the instrument tips become visible on the opposite side of the pedicle. At that point, the surgeon is certain that a 360° dissection around the pedicle has been completed, allowing clip or suture ligation as warranted by the procedure.

Blunt Dissection Probe

Sharp dissection can be risky in laparoscopic procedures, resulting in bleeding and ultimately to conversion to open surgery. As such, many surgeons prefer to perform tissue dissection with electrosurgical equipment. Some electrosurgical devices do lend themselves to dissection, and these will be discussed later. However, 1 inexpensive device that should be among every veterinary surgeon's instrument set is a blunt probe. Most veterinary surgeons prefer reusable, resterilizable equipment for reasons of cost. However, blunt metallic probes lack some of the qualities of their single-use disposable counterparts. The single-use probes feature a flexible plastic shaft and a gauze tip (**Fig. 10**). This gauze tip becomes important when used for blunt dissection along vascular and tubular structures. When the dry gauze tip is placed in a dissection plane and the instrument shaft is twirled with the fingers, loose connective tissue between tissue structures readily separates. An example of such use would be in separating vascular and ureteral structures during laparoscopic nephrectomy. Furthermore, the dissection is further facilitated by, not only twirling the instrument shaft, but also moving the probe tip in the direction of the vessels. Vascular damage is prevented in this fashion. Another clinical example of the utility of a gauze-tipped blunt probe is in detaching the gall bladder from the liver during cholecystectomy. The same twirling method is used, with the probe being spun from the liver edge

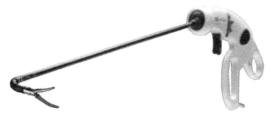

Fig. 9. SILS Maryland dissector: features pivot joint at junction of instrument shaft and handle, which allows 360° of movement arc; locking trigger maintains instrument position. (*Courtesy of* Covidien; with permission. All rights reserved.)

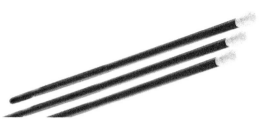

Fig. 10. Cotton-tipped, atraumatic laparoscopic probes. (*Courtesy of* Covidien; with permission. All rights reserved.)

toward the gall bladder. It is the friction caused by the dry gauze that causes the tissue separation. Metallic tipped probes do not allow such dissection because of the lack of friction between the moist tip and the tissue.

Monopolar Pencil Electrode Extensions

Aspiring veterinary laparoscopists are often intimidated and discouraged by the high equipment costs associated with laparoscopy. However, there are a few instances in which existing equipment can be readily adapted for laparoscopic use. One such instance involves the use of monopolar electrosurgery. Most veterinary surgical practices own some form of cautery box, which delivers cutting, coagulating, or blended electrosurgical energy through a monopolar pencil and/or a bipolar forceps. The same monopolar pencil can be readily fitted with an electrode extension to allow insertion through a laparoscopic port and use within the abdomen (**Fig. 11**). Laparoscopic electrode extensions usually have a J-shaped or L-shaped configuration (**Figs. 12** and **13**). This configuration allows the surgeon to lightly hook the tissue with the concave aspect or use the back (convex) side for blunt dissection. Electrosurgical energy is applied in such a way as to weaken the tissue, after which light traction causes the tissue to separate. When practiced judiciously, this is an effective dissection method.

Laparoscopic Aspirator/Lavage with Monopolar Hook

The most common reason for laparoscopic conversion is uncontrolled hemorrhage. Even so, most veterinary surgeons do not make provisions for laparoscopic suction/lavage, at least for routine procedures. When delicate dissection is required, as occurs during adrenalectomy, it is wise to have a suction/lavage system available. The suction/lavage instrument is usually 5 mm in diameter and has a fenestrated tip to allow it to act like a sump pump (**Fig. 14**). Fluids can be readily aspirated without sucking tissue into the instrument tip. Some of these devices have a monopolar pin on the handle, allowing attachment to a monopolar energy source. An extendable wire can be deployed from the instrument end to allow application to a bleeding vessel. It is important to remember that a grounding pad must be applied to the patient in order for this monopolar system to function.

5 mm Miniretractor

Numerous retractor types are available to the veterinary laparoscopist. In many instances, they are too bulky and traumatic to be used for general retraction, especially in limited spaces. To that end, a 5 mm miniretractor may be helpful. The retractor is placed through a 5 mm port, and is extended into a semicircular hook once in the abdomen. This hook is helpful in isolating the cystic arteries and duct during cholecystectomy, as well as in retracting the kidneys during adrenalectomy (**Fig. 15**).

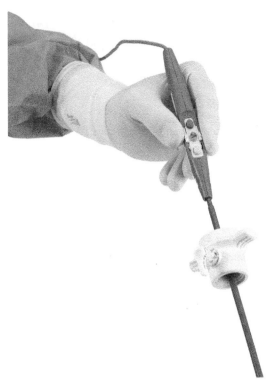

Fig. 11. Monopolar electrode extension: attachment to a conventional electrosurgical pencil allows laparoscopic delivery of monopolar energy; a patient return electrode (*grounding pad*) must be used with this system. (*Courtesy of* Covidien; with permission. All rights reserved.)

Energy-Based Devices

Laparoscopic dissection and hemostasis are most frequently achieved with some form of electrosurgical device. This may include monopolar electrosurgery as described previously or a simple bipolar forceps, which can be plugged into the bipolar side of a standard electrosurgical box. However, newer energy-based devices have been developed in order to minimize surgeon errors associated with inappropriate application with respect to tissue type, quantity of applied energy, or duration of applied energy.

Vessel Sealing Devices

LigaSure

The Ligasure first generation (Medtronic) vessel sealing device (**Fig. 16**) received US Food and Drug Administration (FDA) approval in 1998, but was not used extensively in veterinary surgery until 2007.[17] The generator contains bipolar and Ligasure

Fig. 12. J-shaped monopolar electrode extension. (*Courtesy of* Covidien; with permission. All rights reserved.)

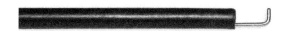

Fig. 13. L-shaped monopolar electrode extension. (*Courtesy of* Covidien; with permission. All rights reserved.)

modules, but no monopolar capability. Initially, laparoscopic spay surgeries presented an ideal application of vessel sealing technology. Ovariectomy and ovariohysterectomy could be performed in a fraction of the time that it would take to perform these procedures with clips or suture. As veterinarians became comfortable with the Ligasure device, numerous other applications were developed. At present, the Ligasure device is no longer manufactured. However, refurbished and used generators are generally available through the manufacturer or medical equipment resellers, respectively.

Enseal tissue sealing device

The Enseal (Ethicon, Somerville, New Jersey) tissue sealing device is similar in operation to the Ligasure device, but with some notable differences. The EnSeal tissue seal is performed as a 1-stage operation in that energy delivery occurs simultaneously with instrument closure and tissue division. The LigaSure device requires that instrument closure, energy activation, and tissue division occur as separate operations. The vascular seal achieved with the Enseal device achieves higher burst pressure and a smaller margin of lateral thermal spread than that of the LigaSure device. Enseal handpieces are available in 5 mm and 12 mm diameters, and some 5 mm versions feature a malleable shaft at the instrument tip. As of this writing, a cordless Enseal device is reported to be in development and may be available in the near future.[18]

Force Triad energy platform (Ligasure, second generation)

The Force Triad (FT) energy platform (**Fig. 17**) was FDA-approved in 2007, but did not enter the veterinary market until around 2010.[19] The FT generator is an all-in-one generator, and includes monopolar, bipolar, and Ligasure technologies. Vessel sealing times are approximately twice as fast as those obtained with the first-generation Ligasure device. The FTd unit features touch-screen controls, which are software upgradeable as new instruments are developed. A dedicated cart gives the FT platform the portability to be moved between operative suites.

One FT handpiece that allows use of all generator modalities in 1 instrument is the LigaSure Advance instrument. The handpiece features a tissue sealing tip, to which is attached a metal projection for monopolar energy delivery. Vessel sealing devices are well-suited to vessel occlusion, but not delicate dissection. The monopolar tip on the device allows the surgeon to perform fine dissection concurrently with tissue sealing, thus minimizing instrument changes and decreasing operative time[20] (**Figs. 18** and **19**).

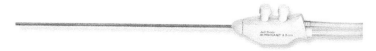

Fig. 14. Laparoscopic suction/irrigation device: often features a monopolar pin connector and delivery wire to coagulate small vessels (*not pictured*). (*Courtesy of* Covidien; with permission. All rights reserved.)

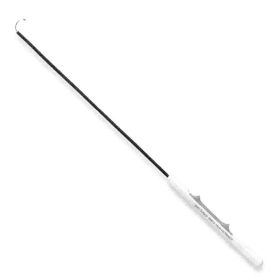

Fig. 15. 5 mm miniretractor. Straight shaft allows easy insertion into cannula; sliding button deploys J-shaped hook. (*Courtesy of* Covidien; with permission. All rights reserved.)

Ultrasonic Energy Devices

Ultrasonic energy devices have been around since the late 1980s. Ultrasonic dissector/coagulators consist of a generator, a transducer, and handpieces that are designed to cut and coagulate tissue. Traditionally, these devices require wired connections from an electrical outlet to the generator, and from the generator to the transducer, which is attached to the handpiece. In 2011, a cordless ultrasonic dissector/coagulator (**Fig. 20**) was developed that housed the ultrasonic generator and transducer within a single instrument. Furthermore, the instrument was only slightly larger than a traditional ultrasonic energy handpiece. This technology is still relatively new to the human surgical market, and as such, fetches a premium price.

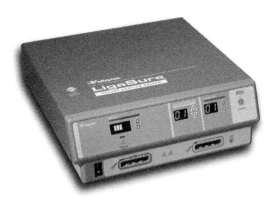

Fig. 16. LigaSure vessel-sealing generator: supplies conventional and specialized bipolar energySure; first generation LigaSure device. (*Courtesy of* Covidien; with permission. All rights reserved.)

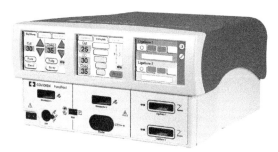

Fig. 17. Force Triad energy platform: supplies monopolar, conventional bipolar, and special-ized bipolar energy; second generation Ligasure device. (*Courtesy of* Covidien; with permis-sion. All rights reserved.)

Although ultrasonic energy devices are excellent dissectors, they have, until recently, lacked the capacity to coagulate vessels as large as those handled by specialized vessel/tissue sealers such as the Enseal and the Ligasure/FT devices. The Harmonic Ace (Ethicon Inc, Somerville, NJ, USA), the long-time ultrasonic surgical market leading product, was recently improved to allow coagulation of vessels up to 7 mm in diameter. This puts it on par with dedicated vessel sealers in sealing large ves-sels. Furthermore, it can be used with the same generator that is used to power the Enseal device. Essentially, one can have it all with this system, although it is not sold directly into the veterinary market.[21]

Laparoscopic Stapling

Laparoscopic endostaplers consist of a loading handle and a disposable loading unit (DLU). The DLU consists of rows of staples of the same size, with or without an inte-grated cutting blade. Two common problems associated with the use of laparoscopic endostaplers are: (1) inconsistent sealing across the staple line due to variable tissue thickness and (2) extrusion of tissue from the stapler jaws during firing. To this end, 2 new stapling technologies have emerged.

Tri-Staple technology
Traditional endostapling DLUs are offered in 30 mm, 45 mm, and 60 mm linear lengths, and 2.0 mm, 2.5 mm, 3.5 mm, and 4.8 mm staple leg lengths. Staples within a given

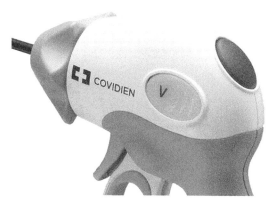

Fig. 18. Advance bipolar sealer/divider with monopolar coagulation/dissector tip: instru-ment controls. (*Courtesy of* Covidien; with permission. All rights reserved.)

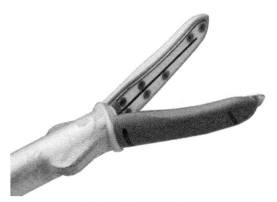

Fig. 19. Advance bipolar sealer/divider with monopolar coagulation/dissector tip: instrument tip showing sealer/divider jaws and monopolar electrode. (*Courtesy of* Covidien; with permission. All rights reserved.)

loading unit are of the same dimension. A new technology was developed that features staples of varying leg length within a single DLU (**Fig. 21**). In the case of a linear stapling/dividing instrument (gastrointestinal anastomosis [GIA] device), the staple row nearest the cut line has staples whose leg lengths are shorter than those in the outer row of staples. This variation in staple leg length from the cut line to the outer row of staples was designed to alleviate the problems noted previously. As the Tri-Staple (TST, Medtronic) cartridge is closed, tissue fluids are directed laterally, causing functional thinning of the tissue to be stapled (**Fig. 22**). Less tissue bulk within the instrument results in less extrusion from the cartridge and anvil ends as the cartridge is closed, staples are formed, and the cutting bar advanced. The overall result is a more consistently reliable stapled line. TST cartridges come in 3 options to address tissue thicknesses, ranging from 0.88 mm up to 3.0 mm.[22]

Two specialized modifications of the TST cartridge have been developed. A curved tip TST DLU is available for use in tight spaces (**Fig. 23**). With this device, a rubber introducer is attached to the cartridge anvil hook to serve as a grasping point to pull the cartridge into firing position. A reinforced TST reload featuring an absorbable staple backing material is also available (**Fig. 24**). This buttress material increases staple

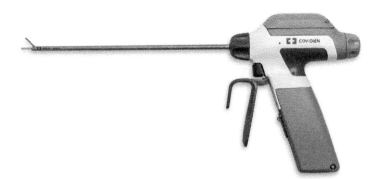

Fig. 20. Sonicision cordless ultrasonic dissector: rechargeable battery, generator, transducer, and dissecting/coagulating tip(s) all contained within 1 handpiece. (*Courtesy of* Covidien; with permission. All rights reserved.)

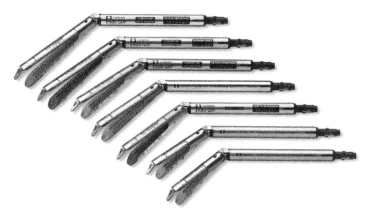

Fig. 21. TST roticulating endostapling cartridges; a wide range of cartridge lengths and variable staple leg lengths allow sealing across a wide range of tissue thicknesses. (*Courtesy of* Covidien; with permission. All rights reserved.)

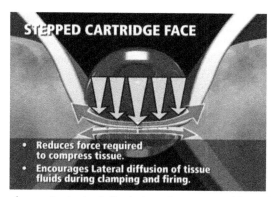

Fig. 22. TST closure forces. As stapler is fired, tissue is compressed laterally, resulting in less tissue extrusion from the end of the staple cartridge. (*Courtesy of* Covidien; with permission. All rights reserved.)

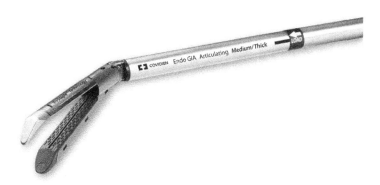

Fig. 23. TST cartridge with curved tip; a rubber introducer attached to tip is used to maneuver cartridge into desired firing position. (*Courtesy of* Covidien; with permission. All rights reserved.)

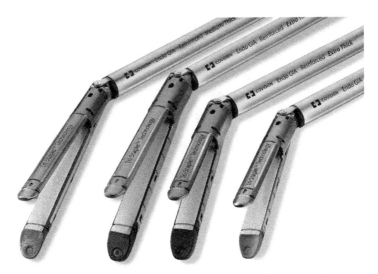

Fig. 24. Reinforced TST reload; absorbable buttress material increases burst pressure and provides improved hemostatic and pneumostatic closure. (*Courtesy of* Covidien; with permission. All rights reserved.)

line burst pressure and provides a more rigorous hemostatic and pneumostatic closure. As such, these specialized TST cartridges are particularly useful in thoracic surgery.

REFERENCES

1. Devitt CM, Cox RE, Hailey JJ. Duration, complications, stress, and pain of open ovariohysterectomy versus a simple method of laparoscopic-assisted ovariohysterectomy in dogs. J Am Vet Med Assoc 2005;227(6):921–7.
2. Dupre G, Fiorbianco V, Skalicky M, et al. Laparoscopic ovariectomy in dogs: comparison between single portal and two-portal access. Vet Surg 2009;38(7):818–24.
3. Doerner J, Fiorbianco V, Dupre G. Intercostal insertion of Veress needle for canine laparoscopic procedures: a cadaver study. Vet Surg 2012;41(3):362–6.
4. Fiorbianco V, Skalicky M, Doerner J, et al. Right intercostal insertion of a Veress needle for laparoscopy in dogs. Vet Surg 2012;41(3):367–73.
5. Whittemore JC, Mitchell A, Hyink S, et al. Diagnostic accuracy of tissue impedance measurement interpretation for correct Veress needle placement in canine cadavers. Vet Surg 2013;42(5):613–22.
6. Minami S, Okamoto Y, Eguchi H, et al. Successful laparoscopy assisted ovariohysterectomy in two dogs with pyometra. J Vet Med Sci 1997;59(9):845–7.
7. Austin B, Lanz OI, Hamilton SM, et al. Laparoscopic ovariohysterectomy in nine dogs. J Am Anim Hosp Assoc 2003;39(4):391–6.
8. Davidson EB, Moll HD, Payton ME. Comparison of laparoscopic ovariohysterectomy and ovariohysterectomy in dogs. Vet Surg 2004;33(1):62–9.
9. Runge JJ, Curcillo PG, King SA, et al. Initial application of reduced port surgery using the single port access technique for laparoscopic canine ovariohysterectomy. Vet Surg 2012;41(7):803–6.
10. Coisman JG, Case JB, Clark ND, et al. Efficacy of decontamination and sterilization of a single-use single-incision laparoscopic surgery port. Am J Vet Res 2013;74(6):934–8.

11. Runge JJ, Mayhew PD. Evaluation of single port access gastropexy and ovariectomy using articulating instruments and angled telescopes in dogs. Vet Surg 2013;42(7):807–13.
12. Villa MT, White LE, Alam M, et al. Barbed sutures: a review of the literature. Plast Reconstr Surg 2008;121(3):102e–8e.
13. Bassi A, Tulandi T. Evaluation of total laparoscopic hysterectomy with and without the use of barbed suture. J Obstet Gynaecol Can 2013;35(8):718–22.
14. Runge JJ, Mayhew P, Rawlings CA. Laparoscopic-assisted and laparoscopic prophylactic gastropexy: indications and techniques. Compend Contin Educ Vet 2009;31(2):E2.
15. Mayhew PD, Brown DC. Prospective evaluation of two intracorporeally sutured prophylactic gastropexy techniques compared with laparoscopic-assisted gastropexy in dogs. Vet Surg 2009;38(6):738–46.
16. Available at: http://www.covidien.com/surgical/products/hand-instruments-and-ligation/endoscopic-suturing-devices. Accessed September 15, 2015.
17. Mayhew PD, Brown DC. Comparison of three techniques for ovarian pedicle hemostasis during laparoscopic-assisted ovariohysterectomy. Vet Surg 2007;36(6):541–7.
18. Available at: http://gb.ethicon.com/healthcare-professionals/products/energy-devices/enseal-g2-superjaw#!overview. Accessed September 15, 2015.
19. Available at: http://www.vet.uga.edu/mis/equipment/energy.php. Accessed September 15, 2015.
20. Available at: http://www.covidien.com/surgical/products/vessel-sealing/laparoscopic-instruments/ligasure-advance-pistol-grip. Accessed September 15, 2015.
21. Available at: http://www.ethicon.com/healthcare-professionals/products/advanced-energy/harmonic/harmonic-ace-plus-seven. Accessed September 15, 2015.
22. Available at: http://www.covidien.com/surgical/products/stapling. Accessed September 15, 2015.

Anesthesia for Endoscopy

Makoto Asakawa, BVSc

KEYWORDS

- Pneumoperitoneum • Gas embolism • One-lung ventilation • V/Q mismatch
- Capnothorax • CO_2

KEY POINTS

- Anesthetists should focus on only anesthetic management and not be distracted by setting up the endoscopic equipment.
- No single anesthetic protocol has proved superior to other protocols for endoscopic surgery.
- Insufflation induces significant cardiovascular and respiratory changes.
- One-lung ventilation devices should be placed with a bronchoscope.

INTRODUCTION

Compared with laparotomy or thoracotomy, endoscopic surgery in human and veterinary patients has been shown to have multiple benefits, including reduction of the stress response, better respiratory function postoperatively, less postoperative pain and discomfort, and shorter stay in hospital.[1–7] Endoscopic surgery has disadvantages, such as limited visualization of the surgical field, longer duration of surgery, pathophysiologic changes caused by insufflation of gas into the abdominal cavity, and difficulty in evaluating the amount of blood loss, but the benefits overcome these disadvantages.[7–9] For these reasons, endoscopic surgery has become popular in veterinary medicine despite equipment costs.

Endoscopic surgery can be classified as an elective procedure or a nonelective procedure. Elective procedures, such as gastropexy and ovariectomy, are usually performed on young healthy patients. Although anesthetic management on these patients seems simple and straightforward, endoscopic surgery can induce significant systemic changes even in healthy patients and may be associated with complications.[8–10]

Patients undergoing nonelective procedures, such as adrenalectomy, cholecystectomy, portosystemic shunt ligation, lung lobectomy, mass biopsy, and liver biopsy, often have comorbidities. These patients have the same or worse systemic changes

Disclosure: The author has nothing to disclose.
Department of Clinical Sciences, Cornell University College of Veterinary Medicine, VMC Box 35, Ithaca, NY 14853-6401, USA
E-mail address: ma273@cornell.edu

compared with healthy patients, and the rate of complications might be higher than in healthy patients. In addition to these concerns associated with endoscopic surgery, patients' comorbidities affect anesthetic management adversely.[11]

Anesthetists must understand the possible systemic changes and complications that are associated with endoscopic surgery before anesthetizing any patient, even a healthy one. Although it is important to know how comorbidities affect anesthetic management, this article focuses only on anesthetic management of patients undergoing endoscopic surgery and specifically on the systemic changes and complications that can occur.

EFFECT OF PNEUMOPERITONEUM

Endoscopic surgery, especially laparoscopic procedures, requires insufflation of a gas such as helium, argon, nitrous oxide, or carbon dioxide (CO_2) into the abdominal cavity to improve visibility of the surgical field.[9,12,13] CO_2 is the gas most commonly used because it has ideal characteristics: it quickly dissolves in blood, so large amounts can be stored in the blood thus reducing the likelihood of CO_2 thromboembolism; CO_2 is quickly eliminated by exhalation through the lungs; there is no anesthetic effect at clinical concentrations; it is noninflammable; and it does not irritate tissues.[8,9,14] Insufflation of the abdominal cavity with any gas produces pneumoperitoneum, and requires special equipment and techniques.

After placement of a needle or first port using a closed technique (Veress needle) or open technique (Hasson technique), gas insufflation is started before placing the next port. Insufflation creates more space between the body wall and abdominal organs, thus reducing the incidence of abdominal organ damage associated with port placement.

As gas insufflation proceeds, intra-abdominal pressure (IAP) increases. IAP is one of the most critical aspects of laparoscopic surgery because increased CO_2 levels and IAP induce hemodynamic and ventilatory changes.[8,9] During insufflation, IAP and gas flow rate should be monitored closely and adjusted as needed to avoid high pressures.

High IAP induces peripheral vasoconstriction and increases arterial blood pressure.[8,9] This vasoconstriction is caused by the release of neurohormonal factors such as vasopressin and catecholamines.[8,15,16] Increased IAP also compresses the abdominal venous system, which reduces return of blood to the heart.[9] These two effects have been shown in human patients to decrease cardiac output by 20% to 42%.[9,17,18] These hemodynamic changes are most likely to occur when IAP is more than 12 mm Hg in dogs.[19]

Increase of IAP displaces the diaphragm cranially, which reduces lung compliance and functional residual capacity (FRC).[8,9] These changes also increase physiologic dead space in the lung because of ventilation and perfusion (V/Q) mismatch. Therefore, increasing minute ventilation is necessary after inducing pneumoperitoneum to prevent hypoventilation or hypoxemia.[9]

When pneumoperitoneum is created by insufflating CO_2, the CO_2 diffuses through the peritoneum and into vessels where it is absorbed by blood; this results in increasing partial pressures of CO_2 in arterial blood ($Paco_2$), which causes acidemia.[8] Usually, the amount of CO_2 taken up through the peritoneum is too small to cause severe acidemia, but, if peritoneal microvascular damage occurs or blood vessels in the peritoneal cavity are lacerated during insertion of the ports or organ manipulation, CO_2 can diffuse directly into the blood, which can induce severe acidemia.[9]

Brain and renal function can also be affected by pneumoperitoneum. There is a direct correlation between cerebral blood flow (CBF) and intracranial pressure (ICP); as CBF increases, so too does ICP. $Paco_2$ is one of the major factors influencing CBF, and an increase of $Paco_2$ increases CBF because of cerebral vascular vasodilation, resulting in increase of ICP.[20] In patients with an intracranial space-occupying mass, increase of ICP caused by high $Paco_2$ associated with CO_2-induced pneumoperitoneum can cause the patient's condition to deteriorate. Despite maintaining $Paco_2$ within the normal range, pneumoperitoneum can increase blood flow in the brain independently and increase ICP.[21,22] For these reasons, if a patient is known to have or is suspected of having an intracranial space-occupying mass, inducing pneumoperitoneum should be avoided.

Renal function can also be affected by pneumoperitoneum. In people, high IAP decreases renal blood flow and glomerular filtration rate.[9] Urine output significantly decreases during insufflation but returns to normal once abdominal pressure returns to normal.[23]

Pneumoperitoneum-induced increases in IAP significantly affect cardiovascular, respiratory, and renal function and can also increase ICP.[8,9,22] Because of these effects, pneumoperitoneum should not be induced in patients with the following conditions: ventricular peritoneal shunts for treating hydrocephalus; hypovolemia; high ICP; renal failure; and tissue or organ damage within the abdominal cavity. For these patients, laparotomy or gasless laparoscopy may be safer than laparoscopy with pneumoperitoneum.

PREOPERATIVE PREPARATION

Patients should be fasted at least 12 hours before anesthesia to prevent regurgitation and aspiration. To avoid dehydration, patients should have access to water until 2 to 3 hours before premedication.

Pneumoperitoneum reduces cardiovascular and respiratory function, so it is important to assess these functions before anesthetizing the patient.[8,9] A thorough history and a full physical examination are essential. If any problem is suspected or found in either system, 3-view chest radiographs and arterial blood gas analysis must be performed to assess anatomic changes and function. For the cardiovascular system, an electrocardiogram (ECG) and echocardiogram should be performed. If the patient has pleural effusion or pneumothorax, fluid or gas must be removed from the chest cavity, and the patient must be able to ventilate on its own without difficulty. If the amount of fluid or gas is significant or reaccumulates quickly, placement of a chest tube should be considered before anesthetizing the patient. Any cardiac diseases should be managed medically and the patient's condition stabilized before surgery unless emergency surgery is required. If the patient has been given cardiac medications, and as long as the patient is stable with the medications, the medications should be continued even on the day of anesthesia. Hemodynamic changes induced by pneumoperitoneum are largely influenced by the patient's volume status, so dehydrated patients must be rehydrated with fluid therapy before anesthesia.[9]

Just before taking the patient to surgery, the urinary bladder must be emptied, because a full bladder may be damaged when inserting a port in the caudal abdomen; it can also interfere with visibility of the surgical field during laparoscopy.

PREMEDICATION, INDUCTION, AND MAINTENANCE AGENTS

The choice of drugs to use for premedication and anesthetic induction of patients undergoing laparoscopic surgery is complicated by 2 important issues: (1) pain, especially in the postoperative period; and (2) potential drug effects on splenic size, specifically splenomegaly. In terms of pain, the type of endoscopic surgery the patient is having influences the pain that is experienced. Endoscopic surgery has been classified as complete or assisted surgery. Complete endoscopic surgery is performed only through instrument ports, but assisted endoscopic surgery requires an additional incision or an extended incision at a port site, the latter often involving extensive stretching of the incision by instruments. Although endoscopic surgery is considered to be less invasive than open surgery, it still causes tissue trauma that stimulates nociceptive receptors and induces the stress response, so patients should receive analgesics perioperatively. The benefits of providing analgesia are many, including smoother anesthetic induction, stabilized anesthetic maintenance, reduction of minimum alveolar concentration of the inhalant anesthetic, and potentially less postoperative pain.[24,25] Opioids, classified as pure mu agonists, partial mu agonists, and agonist-antagonists, have analgesic as well as sedative properties, and they are often used alone or in combination with other drugs for premedication as well as intraoperative and postoperative analgesia.

If the patient is undergoing complete endoscopic surgery, a partial mu agonist such as buprenorphine should provide sufficient analgesia during surgery. However, if the patient is undergoing assisted endoscopic surgery that involves an additional incision or stretching of a port site, and a partial mu agonist may not provide enough analgesia during surgery, and a pure mu agonist, such as hydromorphone, oxymorphone, methadone, or morphine, is preferred for perioperative analgesia. Some pure mu agonists induce nausea and vomiting, which is uncomfortable for the patient and may lead to perioperative aspiration of gastric contents. Fentanyl does not induce nausea, but its half-life is short and its analgesic effect lasts less than 30 minutes after a single bolus. A technique for overcoming the short duration of effect when using fentanyl as a premedicant is to give the drug intravenously (IV) before induction. If the patient has an intravenous catheter or tolerates insertion of an intravenous catheter without sedation, small amounts of fentanyl (3–5 µg/kg) can be given as a premedicant followed by propofol for induction. To ensure adequate analgesia during surgery, a local anesthetic can be infiltrated at the site of port insertion or a fentanyl constant-rate infusion (CRI) (0.2–0.4 µg/kg/min IV) can be administered.

Drug-induced splenomegaly may increase the risk of injury to the enlarged spleen when the Veress needle or port is inserted into the abdomen. Selecting drugs that cause minimal or no splenic enlargement is important and several studies have addressed this issue.[26–28] In one study, significant splenic enlargement was seen after administering acepromazine or thiopental, but not after administering propofol.[26] Another study found that a combination of acepromazine and butorphanol followed by induction with propofol had minimal effect on splenic volume, whereas medetomidine and butorphanol as premedicants followed by ketamine and diazepam for induction were associated with a significant increase in splenic volume.[27] In a more recent study, acepromazine, propofol, and thiopental treatments caused the greatest increase in splenic volume, whereas hydromorphone and dexmedetomidine used in combination as premedicants did not cause a significant change in splenic volume.[28] Taken together, these studies suggest that, for premedication, combinations of acepromazine plus butorphanol, or hydromorphone plus dexmedetomidine followed by induction with propofol are more likely to have little effect on splenic volume. Other concerns may favor some drugs more than others. Thiopental for induction is not appropriate, because it causes significant splenic engorgement.[26,28]

Alpha-2 agonists, such as dexmedetomidine, can be used for endoscopic anesthesia and might help attenuate cardiovascular effects associated with pneumoperitoneum.[29] However, doses typically used for premedication induce significant hemodynamic changes that may not be desirable in patients with cardiac diseases.

Most induction agents, such as propofol, etomidate, and alfaxalone, can be used without problems. However, in addition to its effects on splenic volume, ketamine stimulates the sympathetic nervous system and increases the release of catecholamines.[30,31] Because pneumoperitoneum also increases the release of catecholamines, ketamine may not be the best choice, especially in patients with cardiovascular disease.[9]

High IAP can increase vagal tone; therefore, giving anticholinergics such as glycopyrrolate, or atropine as a part of premedication is appropriate. In addition to IAP, using opioids also increases vagal tone, which makes patients more prone to develop bradycardia during surgery.

Isoflurane and sevoflurane are appropriate to use for a maintenance agent. However, halothane increases the sensitivity of the heart to catecholamines, so should be avoided.[32] Propofol CRI (0.2–0.5 mg/kg/min IV) can be used safely for a maintenance agent in dogs but not in cats.[33]

N_2O is not an ideal anesthetic gas during endoscopic surgery because it diffuses into gas-filled spaces such as the abdominal cavity and thoracic cavity and increases pressure over time. Also, if a gas embolus occurs during surgery, the volume of the embolus is increased dramatically, and N_2O worsens the situation.

Neuromuscular paralytic drugs, such as atracurium (0.1–0.2 mg/kg IV), can be used during surgery to improve relaxation of the abdominal wall. As a result, less IAP is required to achieve adequate visualization of the surgical field and hemodynamic and ventilatory changes associated with pneumoperitoneum may be minimized.[34] Use of neuromuscular paralytics requires the use of a mechanical ventilator and monitoring of cardiopulmonary variables; at the end of surgery the neuromuscular blockade must be reversed.

MONITORING

Induction of pneumoperitoneum and endoscopic maneuvers can adversely affect the patient's cardiopulmonary function.[8,9] For this reason, anesthetists must focus only on anesthesia and must not be distracted by requests to help with endoscopic or other surgical equipment. Changes in the patient's status can occur at any time during and even after endoscopic surgery. Anesthetists must monitor ECG, blood pressure (either invasive or noninvasive), heart rate, body temperature, pulse oximetry, and capnometry. Pneumoperitoneum or manipulation of tissues near the heart can induce cardiac arrhythmias.[9] Therefore, the ECG is important and should be monitored continuously.

For healthy patients, measuring blood pressure every 3 minutes with a noninvasive blood pressure device should be frequent enough to detect problems. Because invasive blood pressure monitoring requires more time and cost and can have its own set of complications, usually it is not necessary for healthy patients. However, if the patient has concurrent cardiac or pulmonary problem, invasive blood pressure monitoring should be performed. Placing an indwelling catheter in the dorsal pedal artery allows direct blood pressure monitoring and facilitates collecting arterial blood gas samples during and after anesthesia.

Arterial blood gas analysis is very important in endoscopic anesthesia. Not only is it helpful to assess pulmonary function, it also provides a rough estimate of alveolar dead space if $Paco_2$ and end-tidal CO_2 (ET_{CO_2}) are compared simultaneously. A sudden increase of alveolar dead space during endoscopic surgery could indicate development of pulmonary embolism, stressing the need to monitor alveolar dead space.[35] Transesophageal echocardiography and pulmonary arterial catheter are also very helpful for detecting gas embolism and monitoring hemodynamic changes. However, it is not necessary in routine endoscopic anesthesia unless the patient has severe cardiac or respiratory disease.

Core body temperature is affected by endoscopic procedures because the gas used for insufflation is at room temperature or cools the patient during insufflation, thus directly cooling abdominal organs; monitoring and supporting body temperature is crucial. Although thoracoscopy does not require insufflation of gas into the thoracic cavity, ambient air does enter the thoracic cavity and reduces esophageal temperature. Therefore, to accurately monitor body temperature the monitor probe should be in the rectum during thoracoscopy and inserted into the esophagus during laparoscopy to obtain accurate core temperature measurements.

Pulse oximetry provides continuous information concerning hemoglobin saturation with oxygen. Because endoscopic procedures depress ventilation, early detection of hypoxemia is important to avoid complications.

$ETco_2$ measures partial pressure of CO_2 (Pco_2) at the end of expiration, which represents Pco_2 in the alveoli. Because alveolar Pco_2 is supposed to be the same as $Paco_2$, $ETco_2$ can be used for estimating $Paco_2$ and ventilatory function. Laparoscopy increases $Paco_2$ because of insufflation of CO_2 and ventilatory depression associated with high IAP.[9] Thoracoscopy also induces pneumothorax, which depresses ventilation. Therefore, monitoring $ETco_2$ to detect hypoventilation is important. In addition, $ETco_2$ guides adjustment of ventilator settings to effectively treat hypoventilation during general anesthesia.

ANESTHETIC MANAGEMENT

If the patient has a cardiopulmonary problem or if it is going to be induced with a drug known to cause hypoventilation or apnea, the patient should be preoxygenated for at least 5 minutes via a mask or using a flow-by technique before induction. If propofol or fentanyl was chosen as a part of induction, it should be administered slowly to avoid side effects such as respiratory arrest, hypotension, or bradycardia. During induction, the anesthetist must monitor at least both heart rate and respiratory rate by palpating pulse and observing chest movement. All patients must be intubated and induced to general anesthesia for endoscopic surgery to support pulmonary function. All monitoring equipment and additional catheters, if necessary, should be placed before moving the patient into the operation room.

Before making incisions for the instrument ports, local anesthetics, such as bupivacaine, should be infiltrated around the surgical sites to provide analgesia. The total amount of bupivacaine should not exceed 2 mg/kg in dogs and 1 mg/kg in cats, which is less than the intravenous toxic dose to prevent the toxic effects of this local anesthetic.[36,37] A liposome encapsulated formulation of bupivacaine has been used in human patients, and produces analgesia lasting up to 72 hours after infiltration.[38,39] No clinical study of this particular formulation has been published in veterinary medicine, but it could be a good alternative to postoperative administration of opioids.

If hydromorphone or methadone was used in premedication, the analgesic effect should last until the end of surgery (4–6 hours). If additional analgesia is necessary, a CRI of either fentanyl or dexmedetomidine can be added to the anesthetic protocol during surgery.

LAPAROSCOPIC SURGERY

Induction of pneumoperitoneum causes an increase in mean arterial pressure and a decrease in cardiac output, usually without altering heart rate.[8,9] If the IAP is less than 12 mm Hg, these hemodynamic changes are not significant.[9] If insufflation is too rapid, significant hemodynamic changes can occur but can be counteracted by making sure the patient is adequately hydrated before inducing the pneumoperitoneum. Giving a bolus of crystalloids (10–20 mL/kg) over 10 to 15 minutes before starting insufflation can minimize these hemodynamic changes, especially if the patient has cardiac disease or is hypovolemic.[9] Induction of pneumoperitoneum should be performed smoothly and slowly.

Insufflation of CO_2 increases $Paco_2$ because of absorption through the abdominal peritoneum.[8] This increase in $Paco_2$ can be normalized by adjusting ventilator settings to increase minute ventilation. However, if the ventilator setting adversely affects cardiovascular function and does not normalize $Paco_2$, maintaining $Paco_2$ around 50 mm Hg is acceptable in most patients as long as blood pH is higher than 7.3. An exception is patients with intracranial disease, because hypercapnia increases CBF and, as a result, increases ICP. In patients with intracranial disease, normocapnia must be maintained throughout the anesthetic period to prevent brain injury.

Increased IAP shifts the diaphragm cranially and decreases FRC and compliance of the lung.[8,9] Because these changes adversely affect ventilatory function, patients should be mechanically ventilated. Adjusting ventilator settings to normalize $Paco_2$ can be challenging with these respiratory changes, especially the reduced lung compliance. Usually a larger tidal volume setting and a slower than normal respiratory frequency provide better ventilation with these pulmonary changes than do small tidal volumes and a fast rate.[9] In some patients, it is necessary to apply a small amount of positive end-expiratory pressure (PEEP), such as 5 cm H_2O, to prevent atelectasis.[40]

Although rare, gas embolism can occur during pneumoperitoneum.[9] Usually gas absorption from the abdominal cavity through the peritoneum is minimal. However, if the peritoneum is damaged because of surgical manipulation or the patient develops subcutaneous emphysema caused by gas insufflation, the amount of gas absorbed can become significant and may induce gas embolism.[10] If a gas embolus develops, $ETco_2$ decreases suddenly because of high V/Q ratio even though the ventilator setting has not been changed.[31] In addition to $ETco_2$ changes, blood pressure and Spo_2 may decrease at the same time, but depend on the size of the embolus.

Making a diagnosis of gas embolism is not easy and requires chest radiographs, CT examination with angiography, or the use of a transesophageal echocardiography; however, these modalities may not be available or may take time to acquire. Gas embolism can be fatal. In the absence of a clear diagnosis, anesthetists must start appropriate treatments or prevent worsening of the situation if any of the signs discussed earlier are seen. Gas insufflation must be promptly discontinued, and the abdomen deflated as soon as possible. The patient should be positioned in the Trendelenburg position (tilt head down with patient in dorsal recumbency) to prevent further gas movement toward the heart.[9] If the symptoms are severe, such as adversely affecting cardiac output, inserting a central venous catheter to the level of the right heart and aspirating the gas may remove the embolus.[41] If the patient is in an emergency condition and has minimal cardiac output, shaking the patient's body may decrease the size of the gas embolus and may help to reestablish blood flow through the heart and pulmonary artery.[42] Once the major gas embolus is cleared, small gas emboli dissolve into the blood quickly, especially if the gas used for insufflation was CO_2.

Another complication that may occur during pneumoperitoneum is pneumothorax, which is often caused by accidental diaphragmatic injury. If CO_2 was used for insufflation and the patient developed pneumothorax, it is called capnothorax, which increases $ETco_2$ and inspiratory airway pressure. Subcutaneous emphysema also increases $ETco_2$; an easy means for distinguishing between capnothorax and subcutaneous emphysema during pneumoperitoneum is to assess inspiratory airway pressure. If the inspiratory airway pressure has increased, it is less likely that the patient has subcutaneous emphysema.[9] If a capnothorax is suspected, gas insufflation must be discontinued immediately and then careful chest auscultation and chest radiograph should be performed. Capnothorax resolves quickly (30–60 minutes) because CO_2 has high solubility in blood and is absorbed by the blood once insufflation is discontinued.[43] When a patient develops capnothorax during a procedure, it may require ventilatory support, such as applying PEEP or increasing minute ventilation until the capnothorax resolves. Thoracocentesis should be avoided unless the patient develops severe clinical signs, because the capnothorax resolves quickly without treatment.[43] As long as the patient is stable and has adequate ventilatory function at the end of anesthesia, such as $Paco_2$ less than 50 mm Hg and Spo_2 more than 95%, the patient can recover normally with careful respiratory monitoring.

Subcutaneous emphysema can develop during pneumoperitoneum and usually is associated with accidental extraperitoneal insufflation.[9] If the subcutaneous emphysema is caused by CO_2 insufflation, there is an increase in $ETco_2$ without a change in airway pressure.[9] As for CO_2-induced pneumothorax, CO_2 insufflation should be discontinued immediately and the patient provided ventilatory support until most of the emphysema is absorbed. These treatments are adequate in most cases.

The arrhythmia associated with pneumoperitoneum or manipulation of abdominal organs is usually bradyarrhythmia caused by of vagal stimulation.[44] If a patient develops hypotension caused by bradyarrhythmia, an anticholinergic agent (glycopyrrolate, 0.02 mg/kg IV) should be administered. However, anticholinergic treatment is not necessary for most bradyarrhythmias when the blood pressure is normal. If tachyarrhythmia develops because of catecholamine release, such as that associated with adrenalectomy, a short-acting β-blocker (esmolol, 0.25–0.5 mg/kg IV slowly) or lidocaine (2 mg/kg IV) can be administered depending on the type of tachyarrhythmia.

If the surgical procedure requires that the table be tilted, as for ovariectomy, tilting must be slow to avoid sudden hemodynamic and respiratory changes.[45] After changing patient position, if the Spo_2 decreases without a change in $ETco_2$, or $ETco_2$ suddenly diminishes, it could be caused by dislocation of the endotracheal tube or disconnection of the endotracheal tube from the breathing circuit. Whenever a change has occurred in patient position and if any airway problem occurs, the anesthetist must check depth of anesthesia, airway patency, and connection of endotracheal tube to the breathing circuit.

THORACOSCOPIC SURGERY

After placing the introducer, a small amount of gas is insufflated into the thoracic cavity or room air is used to create pneumothorax before placing the next port. Pneumothorax reduces the size of the lung on the surgical side and creates a space between chest wall and lung, which reduces the risk of lung puncture or laceration associated with inserting an additional port. This pneumothorax also improves visualization of the intrathoracic structures during the surgical procedure. Unlike laparoscopy, thoracoscopic procedures are performed without pressurized insufflation because the chest cavity is less compliant than the abdominal cavity and because of the severe effects that increased intrathoracic pressure would have on both ventilation and circulation.

In addition to purposely inducing pneumothorax, 1-lung ventilation (OLV) is often performed to obtain maximum visibility during surgery. OLV is induced by using a special endotracheal tube or a bronchial blocker. These devices occlude 1 bronchus, which results in cessation of ventilation of the occluded lung while the other lung remains normally ventilated. Although the blocked side of the lung has no ventilation, it is still perfused by the pulmonary circulation, which carries away gas from alveoli in the occluded lung. As a result, the occluded lung collapses within a few minutes because of gas absorption by pulmonary circulation, especially when greater than 95% oxygen is used as the carrier gas for the inhalant anesthetic agent. Collapsing the lung on the operative side provides a much better surgical field than that provided by a pneumothorax.

The special endotracheal tube, a double-lumen endobronchial tube (**Fig. 1**), has 1 short tube and 1 longer tube and 2 cuffs. The end of the longer tube fits into the left bronchus and the shorter tube is in the trachea. Inflating the cuffs allows positive pressure ventilation of both the right and left lungs. The cuff on the longer end seals only the left bronchus, which isolates the left lung from the right lung. If the shorter tube is occluded, the right lung will not be ventilated, whereas the left lung is ventilated. In contrast, if the longer tube is occluded and not the shorter tube, the right lung is ventilated.

Double-lumen endotracheal tubes are made for human patients, and people have shorter tracheas compared with dogs. If the veterinary patient weighs more than 20 kg, even the longer of the two tubes may not extend to the bronchus. Also, a small-diameter tube is not available, so these tubes are too big for use in small patients such as shih tzu dogs. Use of this endotracheal tube is limited by its circumference and length. If a double-lumen endobronchial tube is appropriate for a given patient, it is important to choose a double-lumen tube with a longer tube that fits into the left bronchus. Longer tubes that fit into the right bronchus of humans do not fit in dogs because of anatomic differences.

An endobronchial blocker (also called bronchial blocker) is also used for OLV during thoracoscopy. The endobronchial blocker (**Fig. 2**) is inserted through an endotracheal tube to either the right or left bronchus; once in position, the cuff on the blocker is inflated, thus occluding the selected bronchus. This device has been used in veterinary medicine more commonly than double-lumen endotracheal tubes because they are not limited by size or length. Correct positioning of either device can be ascertained by auscultation (blind technique); however, the malpositioning rate is high; using a bronchoscope to confirm correct placement is highly recommended.[46]

OLV decreases V/Q ratio (only 1 side of the lung ventilated and blood flow perfuses both side) and worsens pulmonary gas exchange. Although OLV has adequate gas

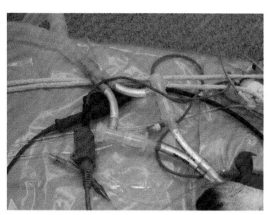

Fig. 1. Double-lumen endobronchial tube is connected to the rebreathing circuit (*left*). The blue tube is marked with the word "Bronchial", indicating that it is the longer side.

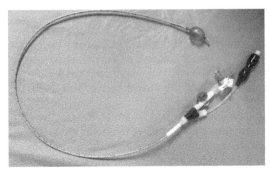

Fig. 2. Endobronchial blocker has a cuff at the near end of the blocker to occlude the bron-chus (*top right*).

exchange to remove CO_2, it may not be enough to maintain oxygenation. If a patient has cardiac or respiratory disease, OLV may not be appropriate, because these patients may not be able to tolerate the change in pulmonary function. After starting OLV, Spo_2 must be monitored closely, and if there is any question or concern about the Spo_2 reading, arterial blood gas analysis should be performed. If hypoxemia develops, appropriate action must be taken as soon as possible. If hypoxemia is severe, OLV must be discontinued immediately. If hypoxemia is mild to moderate, altering ventilator settings to high frequency and low tidal volume may improve oxygenation. If the patient is in lateral recumbency and the dependent lung has normal ventilation, application of the PEEP may correct the hypoxemia. If the double-lumen tube or the bronchial blocker are not available, cannot be inserted, or the patient cannot tolerate OLV, then low-volume and high-frequency ventilator settings may provide a suitable surgical field.

Inducing pneumothorax or directly stimulating the heart may induce cardiac arrhythmias, particularly during pericardiectomy. The ECG must be monitored, and arrhythmias caused by direct stimulation usually respond well to a lidocaine bolus (2 mg/kg in dogs).

Once surgery has been completed, the pneumothorax must be corrected before recovering the patient. The following maneuver is usually adequate for most patients. While the surgeon closes the last surgical site, the anesthetist maximally inflates the lung by squeezing the reservoir bag. This maneuver can eliminate most of the gas from the chest cavity. If this maneuver does not remove most of the gas from the chest cavity or if there is any concern about the accumulation of fluid or gas in the chest cavity during the recovery period, a chest tube should be inserted before recovering the patient.

If the patient undergoes a complete endoscopic procedure, not an assisted endoscopic procedure, then postoperative pain is usually minimal because the patient has only a few centimeter-long incisions. In most cases, a combination of a nonsteroidal antiinflammatory drug (NSAID) and a weak opioid (tramadol) provides enough postoperative analgesia.

If the patient has had assisted endoscopic surgery, one of the incisions is usually more than 5 cm in length and is well stretched during surgery. In this situation, the patient can have significant postoperative pain. A combination of an NSAID and a potent opioid, such as hydromorphone, oxymorphone, or methadone, is administered at least for the first 12 to 24 hours after surgery, and then switching to a weak opioid should provide enough postoperative analgesia.

RECOVERY

Despite better pulmonary function following endoscopic surgery than following laparotomy, before extubating a patient its pulmonary function must be evaluated to ascertain that it is adequate. Evaluation of pulmonary function includes oxygenation and ventilatory function. Testing oxygenation can be done with an oxygen challenge test using either a pulse oximeter or blood gas analysis. This test evaluates the patient's arterial oxygen saturation level while it is breathing room air (fraction of inspired oxygen [Fio_2], 21%) during anesthetic recovery; this gives an indication as to what the patient's oxygenation will be after recovery. Reducing Fio_2 from greater than 95% can be achieved either by disconnecting the endotracheal tube from the breathing circuit or by decreasing Fio_2 using air and oxygen blender on the anesthesia machine, if available. While the patient is breathing room air, Spo_2 is monitored with the pulse oximeter; if Spo_2 decreases to less than 92%, the test must be stopped and the patient allowed to breathe gas with an Fio_2 greater than 50%. If the patient can maintain Spo_2 more than 93% while breathing room air for 3 to 5 minutes, most likely the patient can be recovered without oxygen support. However, if the patient cannot maintain oxygenation, it should be evaluated to determine what factors may be decreasing oxygenation, such as pain, pneumothorax(capnothorax), pneumoperitoneum, dislocation of endotracheal tube, pulmonary embolism, atelectasis, or respiratory depression. If necessary, providing oxygen supplementation after recovery should be considered.

$ETco_2$ should be monitored to check that the patient is adequately ventilating. If the patient cannot maintain $ETco_2$ less than 50 mm Hg, it must be evaluated for factors that can cause hypoventilation or airway obstruction. During anesthetic recovery, respiratory depression often occurs because of too much analgesic or sedative drugs. If a drug is suspected of causing respiratory depression, it should be reversed if possible, and reversal must be done carefully so as not to reverse the salutary effects (eg, analgesia) of the drug.

Spo_2 and $ETco_2$ should be measured early in the recovery period so that the anesthetist is aware of what these variables are after extubation. Once the patient becomes too awake to keep it intubated, these variables often are difficult to monitor and may not be reliable. Knowing how these variables are trending before extubation gives the anesthetist confidence in assessing and managing the patient's recovery. The cardiovascular system must be monitored during recovery, including ECG, heart rate, and blood pressure. Again, these variables help the anesthetist assess the patient's recovery.

If the patient has cardiac disease, monitoring should extend for at least 24 hours after surgery. After general anesthesia, crackles or increased lung sounds are usually auscultated because of intubation and dry air stimulating mucus production in the airways. If the anesthetist has any concern regarding pulmonary edema, auscultation should not be the single diagnostic tool and a chest radiograph should be taken.

SUMMARY

Anesthesia for endoscopic surgery can be challenging depending on surgical manipulations and patient comorbidity. Anesthetists must understand the possible systemic changes and complications that are associated with endoscopic surgery. Pneumoperitoneum induces vasoconstriction and reduces cardiac output, as well as decreasing FRC in the cardiopulmonary system. Both hypoventilation caused by the thoracoscopic procedure and CO_2 insufflation increase $Paco_2$. To prevent the problems associated with high $Paco_2$, monitoring of $ETco_2$ and capability of positive pressure ventilation, which requires intubation, are crucial during endoscopic surgery. Any sudden change of ET_{CO_2} should be monitored closely because this could indicate development of complications. Endoscopic surgery should be a less invasive procedure; however, providing appropriate analgesia remains necessary.

ACKNOWLEDGMENTS

John W. Ludders.

REFERENCES

1. Haque Z, Rahman M, Siddique MA, et al. Metabolic and stress responses of the body to trauma: produced by the laparoscopic and open cholecystectomy. Mymensingh Med J 2004;13:48–52.
2. Lee JY, Kim MC. Comparison of oxidative stress status in dogs undergoing laparoscopic and open ovariectomy. J Vet Med Sci 2014;76:273–6.
3. Ravimohan SM, Kaman L, Jindal R, et al. Postoperative pulmonary function in laparoscopic versus open cholecystectomy: prospective, comparative study. Indian J Gastroenterol 2005;24:6–8.
4. Joris JL, Hinque VL, Laurent PE, et al. Pulmonary function and pain after gastroplasty performed via laparotomy or laparoscopy in morbidly obese patients. Br J Anaesth 1998;80:283–8.
5. Stevens HP, van de Berg M, Ruseler CH, et al. Clinical and financial aspects of cholecystectomy: laparoscopic versus open technique. World J Surg 1997;21:91–6.
6. Ros A, Gustafsson L, Krook H, et al. Laparoscopic cholecystectomy versus minilaparotomy cholecystectomy: a prospective, randomized, single-blind study. Ann Surg 2001;234:741–9.
7. Arulpragasam SP, Case JB, Ellison GW. Evaluation of costs and time required for laparoscopic-assisted versus open cystotomy for urinary cystolith removal in dogs: 43 cases (2009-2012). J Am Vet Med Assoc 2013;243:703–8.
8. Safran DB, Orlando R 3rd. Physiologic effects of pneumoperitoneum. Am J Surg 1994;167:281–6.
9. Gutt CN, Oniu T, Mehrabi A, et al. Circulatory and respiratory complications of carbon dioxide insufflation. Dig Surg 2004;21:95–105.
10. Fors D, Eiriksson K, Arvidsson D, et al. Gas embolism during laparoscopic liver resection in a pig model: frequency and severity. Br J Anaesth 2010;105:282–8.
11. Bille C, Auvigne V, Libermann S, et al. Risk of anaesthetic mortality in dogs and cats: an observational cohort study of 3546 cases. Vet Anaesth Analg 2012;39:59–68.
12. Gupta A, Watson DI, Ellis T, et al. Tumour implantation following laparoscopy using different insufflation gases. ANZ J Surg 2002;72:254–7.
13. Wong YT, Shah PC, Birkett DH, et al. Peritoneal pH during laparoscopy is dependent on ambient gas environment: helium and nitrous oxide do not cause peritoneal acidosis. Surg Endosc 2005;19:60–4.
14. Richter S, Hückstädt T, Aksakal D, et al. Embolism risk analysis–helium versus carbon dioxide. J Laparoendosc Adv Surg Tech A 2012;22:824–9.
15. Wahba RW, Béïque F, Kleiman SJ. Cardiopulmonary function and laparoscopic cholecystectomy. Can J Anaesth 1995;42:51–63.

16. Neudecker J, Sauerland S, Neugebauer E, et al. The European Association for Endoscopic Surgery clinical practice guideline on the pneumoperitoneum for laparoscopic surgery. Surg Endosc 2002;16:1121–43.
17. Johannsen G, Andersen M, Juhl B. The effect of general anaesthesia on the haemodynamic events during laparoscopy with CO_2-insufflation. Acta Anaesthesiol Scand 1989;33:132–6.
18. Hirvonen EA, Nuutinen LS, Kauko M. Hemodynamic changes due to Trendelenburg positioning and pneumoperitoneum during laparoscopic hysterectomy. Acta Anaesthesiol Scand 1995;39:949–55.
19. Ishizaki Y, Bandai Y, Shimomura K, et al. Safe intraabdominal pressure of carbon dioxide pneumoperitoneum during laparoscopic surgery. Surgery 1993;114: 549–54.
20. Mikhail MS, Murray MJ, Morgan GE. Neurophysiology & anesthesia. In: Mikhail MS, Murray MJ, Morgan GE, editors. Clinical anesthesiology. 3rd edition. New York: Lange Medical Books; 2002. p. 552–66.
21. Schöb OM, Allen DC, Benzel E, et al. A comparison of the pathophysiologic effects of carbon dioxide, nitrous oxide, and helium pneumoperitoneum on intracranial pressure. Am J Surg 1996;172:248–53.
22. Josephs LG, Este-McDonald JR, Birkett DH, et al. Diagnostic laparoscopy increases intracranial pressure. J Trauma 1994;36:815–8.
23. Chiu AW, Chang LS, Birkett DH, et al. The impact of pneumoperitoneum, pneumoretroperitoneum, and gasless laparoscopy on the systemic and renal hemodynamics. J Am Coll Surg 1995;181:397–406.
24. Machado CE, Dyson DH, Grant Maxie M. Effects of oxymorphone and hydromorphone on the minimum alveolar concentration of isoflurane in dogs. Vet Anaesth Analg 2006;33:70–7.
25. Bufalari A, Maggio C, Cerasoli I, et al. Preemptive carprofen for peri-operative analgesia in dogs undergoing tibial plateau leveling osteotomy (TPLO): a prospective, randomized, blinded, placebo controlled clinical trial. Schweiz Arch Tierheilkd 2012;154:105–11.
26. O'Brien RT, Waller KR 3rd, Osgood TL. Sonographic features of drug-induced splenic congestion. Vet Radiol Ultrasound 2004;45:225–7.
27. Wilson DV, Evans AT, Carpenter RA, et al. The effect of four anesthetic protocols on splenic size in dogs. Vet Anaesth Analg 2004;31:102–8.
28. Baldo CF, Garcia-Pereira FL, Nelson NC, et al. Effects of anesthetic drugs on canine splenic volume determined via computed tomography. Am J Vet Res 2012;73:1715–9.
29. Aho M, Scheinin M, Lehtinen AM, et al. Intramuscularly administered dexmedetomidine attenuates hemodynamic and stress hormone responses to gynecologic laparoscopy. Anesth Analg 1992;75:932–9.
30. Ambrisko TD, Hikasa Y, Sato K. Influence of medetomidine on stress-related neurohormonal and metabolic effects caused by butorphanol, fentanyl, and ketamine administration in dogs. Am J Vet Res 2005;66:406–12.
31. Duncan C. Carbon dioxide embolism during laparoscopy: a case report. AANA J 1992;60:139–44.
32. Hikasa Y, Okabe C, Takase K, et al. Ventricular arrhythmogenic dose of adrenaline during sevoflurane, isoflurane, and halothane anaesthesia either with or without ketamine or thiopentone in cats. Res Vet Sci 1996;60:134–7.
33. Andress JL, Day TK, Day D. The effects of consecutive day propofol anesthesia on feline red blood cells. Vet Surg 1995;24:277–82.

34. Madsen MV, Staehr-Rye AK, Gätke MR, et al. Neuromuscular blockade for opti-mising surgical conditions during abdominal and gynaecological surgery: a sys-tematic review. Acta Anaesthesiol Scand 2015;59:1–16.

35. Staffieri F, Lacitignola L, De Siena R, et al. A case of spontaneous venous embo-lism with carbon dioxide during laparoscopic surgery in a pig. Vet Anaesth Analg 2007;34:63–6.

36. Feldman HS, Arthur GR, Covino BG. Comparative systemic toxicity of convulsant and supraconvulsant doses of intravenous ropivacaine, bupivacaine, and lido-caine in the conscious dog. Anesth Analg 1989;69:794–801.

37. Skarda RT, Tranquilli WJ. Local anesthetics. In: Tranquilli WJ, Thurmon JC, Grimm KA, editors. Lumb & Jones veterinary anesthesia and analgesia. 4th edi-tion. Ames (IA): Blackwell Publishing; 2007. p. 395–418.

38. Feierman DE, Kronenfeld M, Gupta PM, et al. Liposomal bupivacaine infiltration into the transversus abdominis plane for postsurgical analgesia in open abdom-inal umbilical hernia repair: results from a cohort of 13 patients. J Pain Res 2014; 16:477–82.

39. Owen RT. Bupivacaine liposome injectable suspension: a new approach to post-surgical pain. Drugs Today (Barc) 2013;49:475–82.

40. Russo A, Di Stasio E, Scagliusi A, et al. Positive end-expiratory pressure during laparoscopy: cardiac and respiratory effects. J Clin Anesth 2013;25:314–20.

41. Burcharth J, Burgdorf S, Lolle I, et al. Successful resuscitation after carbon diox-ide embolism during laparoscopy. Surg Laparosc Endosc Percutan Tech 2012; 22:164–7.

42. Liska WD, Poteet BA. Pulmonary embolism associated with canine total hip replacement. Vet Surg 2003;32:178–86.

43. Joris JL. Anesthesia for laparoscopic surgery. In: Miller RD, editor. Miller's anes-thesia. 6th edition. Philadelphia: Elsevier; 2005. p. 2285–306.

44. Myles PS. Bradyarrhythmias and laparoscopy: a prospective study of heart rate changes with laparoscopy. Aust N Z J Obstet Gynaecol 1991;31:171–3.

45. Rist M, Hemmerling TM, Rauh R, et al. Influence of pneumoperitoneum and pa-tient positioning on preload and splanchnic blood volume in laparoscopic sur-gery of the lower abdomen. J Clin Anesth 2001;13:244–9.

46. Benumof JL. The position of a double-lumen tube should be routinely determined by fiberoptic bronchoscopy. J Cardiothorac Vasc Anesth 1993;7:513–4.

Laparoscopic-Assisted Surgical Procedures

Michele A. Steffey, DVM

KEYWORDS

- Laparoscopy • Minimally invasive • Biopsy • Cystotomy • Gastropexy
- Intestinal surgery • Urinary surgery • Reproductive surgery

KEY POINTS

- Laparoscopic-assisted procedures are an excellent alternative to open celiotomy for diagnostic sampling and certain therapeutic interventions in dogs and cats.
- Laparoscopic-assisted procedures allow a balance between the improved patient recoveries often associated with smaller incisions and the need for appropriate visualization of visceral organs/identification of lesions.
- The organ systems of small animal veterinary patients that are most commonly approached using laparoscopic-assisted procedures include the urinary bladder, the gastrointestinal tract, and the reproductive tracts.
- Procedure-specific morbidities and patient selection should be considered when choosing between assisted laparoscopic and open approaches.
- Like many minimally invasive procedures, there is an individual learning curve for each type of procedure.

INTRODUCTION

Minimally invasive surgery is adopted in veterinary medicine with increasing frequency, and with a wider selection of described procedures. Overall, the benefits of making surgical interventions less invasive include reduced patient morbidity, shortened durations of hospitalization, reduced wound contamination and breakdown, and shorter patient recovery periods.[1] Although many laparoscopic procedures are performed fully intracorporeally, laparoscopic-assisted (LA) procedures offer several benefits. An LA procedure maintains the positive minimally invasive attributes of laparoscopic surgery but may reduce the complexity of certain procedures by allowing challenging maneuvers to be performed outside the peritoneal cavity. Exteriorization of hollow visceral organs also reduces the potential for spillage of luminal contents

The author has nothing to disclose.
Department of Surgical and Radiological Sciences, School of Veterinary Medicine, University of California Davis, 1 Shields Avenue, Davis, CA 95616, USA
E-mail address: masteffey@ucdavis.edu

Vet Clin Small Anim 46 (2016) 45–61
http://dx.doi.org/10.1016/j.cvsm.2015.07.002
0195-5616/16/$ – see front matter

and contamination of the peritoneal cavity and allows for collection of high-quality biopsy samples from multiple sites. Laparoscopic equipment is increasingly available to the veterinary practitioner, and the benefits of LA surgery combined with technical similarity of the end procedure to many open surgical procedures that are already familiar to many veterinarians are causing LA procedures to become more routine and useful in a variety of practice settings.

Instrumentation and principles of minimally invasive abdominal surgery are well covered elsewhere,[2–4] and this article assumes a basic understanding of laparoscopic principles and instrumentation. The minimal instrumentation required for LA procedures includes a laparoscope, a video-imaging system, a gas insufflator, and laparoscopic instruments including grasping forceps (laparoscopic Babcock forceps, laparoscopic Kelly forceps), and a blunt palpation probe. Useful, but not strictly essential, equipment for LA procedures includes a table that allows the patient to be tilted in lateral and craniocaudal directions, expanded laparoscopic instrumentation, and hemostatic devices such as laparoscopic clip appliers, electrocautery, or vessel-sealing devices (eg, LigaSure [Valleylab Inc, Boulder, CO], the Enseal [SurgRX Inc, Redwood City, CA], and the Harmonic Scalpel [Ethicon Endosurgery Inc, Cincinnati, OH]). A study comparing the use of extracorporeal sutures, laparoscopic clips, and a bipolar vessel-sealing device for ovarian pedicle ligation found that the bipolar vessel-sealing device was associated with significantly shorter surgical times and a lower incidence of hemorrhage from the ovarian pedicle[5]; therefore, if the operating surgeon intends to offer LA ovariohysterectomy on a regular basis, investment in a vessel-sealing device is recommended.

INDICATIONS/CONTRAINDICATIONS

The general indication for LA procedures revolves around circumstances in which minimally invasive visual inspection of the abdominal cavity and surgical intervention/biopsy of hollow viscera, or larger, mobile abdominal viscera are desired. An LA procedure allows for exteriorization of the organ in question outside the abdominal cavity for dissection or suturing, which may reduce the need for specialized equipment and limit potential peritoneal contamination from an incised hollow viscus (intestines, urinary bladder).

General contraindications for LA procedures can include:

- Hemoabdomen
- Septic peritonitis
- Peritoneal adhesions
- Diaphragmatic hernia

GENERAL PATIENT CONSIDERATIONS AND POSITIONING FOR LAPAROSCOPIC-ASSISTED TECHNIQUES

As for any minimally invasive procedure, the operating surgeon should be prepared to convert to an open surgical procedure if either an intraoperative complication occurs that requires open access to correct or the minimally invasive approach does not allow the procedure to be completed as planned. For the procedures described here, the patient is usually placed in dorsal recumbency as for an open celiotomy. A tilt-table may be beneficial to allow for Trendelenburg, reverse Trendelenburg, or laterally rotated positioning if useful; alternatively, sandbags may be used to prop the patient at the desired angle, depending on the goals of the procedure. The ventral abdomen should be clipped widely as for an open surgical procedure, and the patient should be aseptically prepared in the standard manner. The patient should be well secured to the operating table to avoid complications with alterations in positioning. Sterile drapes should be placed to allow for easy conversion to an open celiotomy should the need arise, and the sterile surgical instrumentation required for an open abdominal procedure should be ready on the table. Nonemergent reasons that conversion may be required include previous surgery resulting in adhesions that do not allow the organ of interest to be safely exteriorized, patient body condition that precludes adequate visualization of the desired structure(s), or surgeon experience.

In most situations, pneumoperitoneum of 8 to 12 mm Hg is required to generate sufficient operating space within the peritoneal cavity, which may be established by one of several methods according to the preference of the operating surgeon. In 1 approach, after a small (1-cm) skin incision, pneumoperitoneum is introduced by initial placement of, and CO_2 insufflation through, a Veress needle introduced through the linea alba. After pneumoperitoneum reaches the desired pressure, a trocar cannula combined portal is carefully placed through the abdominal wall, most commonly through the linea alba. Because the downward pressure required to place the trocar cannula with this method can deform the body toward the viscera and visualization of the viscera is not yet possible, some surgeons place stay sutures in the linea near the site of portal placement to enable upward traction during this procedure and minimize potential inadvertent contact with the viscera. A modified version of this technique with the Veress needle placed through the last palpable intercostal space has been described, and was demonstrated to facilitate pneumoperitoneum with few consequential complications.[6] In a modified Hasson technique, a 1-cm skin incision is made in the desired site of portal placement. Blunt dissection to the linea alba is followed by a small 3-mm to 4-mm stab incision penetrating the peritoneal cavity. Penetration is confirmed by observation of intra-abdominal fat or omentum before inserting the 6-mm trocar cannula. Once the cannula has engaged with the body wall, the laparoscope may be partially inserted into the cannula to allow visualization as the surgeon continues to advance the cannula and minimize the risk of iatrogenic damage to underlying viscera. Once it is certain that the cannula has advanced into the peritoneal cavity and is not tracking between muscle layers of the abdominal wall, the gas insufflator tubing may be connected, and insufflation to the desired pressure commenced. In most cases, this initial portal placement is performed in a subumbilical location, regardless of method. Careful planning of portal placement is needed, regardless of the chosen method of establishing pneumoperitoneum. The modified Hasson and Veress needle techniques have been described in greater detail elsewhere.[6,7]

Because organs and specimens are generally exteriorized from the abdominal cavity in LA procedures, protection of wound edges and minimizing tissue trauma are important considerations. Placement of an Alexis wound retractor device (Applied Medical, Rancho Santa Margarita, CA) can facilitate optimizing exposure and minimize incision length. These devices are now available in a wide variety of sizes (X-small [2-cm to 4-cm incisions] to XX-large [11-cm to 17-cm incisions]), allowing exteriorization of several organs.

LAPAROSCOPIC-ASSISTED PROCEDURES OF THE URINARY BLADDER

Procedures of the lower urinary tract that lend themselves to an LA approach include LA cystotomy, LA cystolith removal, LA cystopexy, LA tube cystostomy, and LA urinary bladder polyp resections. The operating time required for LA cystotomy has been shown to be approximately 30% longer than open cystotomy, with a higher operating cost, but it was also associated with reduced injectable analgesic use compared with open cystotomy in a retrospective case series of dogs and is considered an acceptable minimally invasive alternative to open cystotomy.[8]

Patient Preparation and Positioning

Once anesthetized, the patient is placed in dorsal recumbency. For access to the urinary bladder, a mild Trendelenburg position (5°–10° less than horizontal) may allow the urinary bladder to fall as cranially as possible and may minimize encroachment by cranial abdominal viscera. If possible, the patient should be clipped and prepared to allow access to the urethral orifice for intraoperative catheterization and flushing.

Approach

Pneumoperitoneum may be established by either Veress needle placement or the open (Hasson) technique according to the preferences of the operating surgeon. The general technique for LA cystotomy for these procedures includes insertion of a 6-mm trocar cannula at the level of, or just slightly caudal to, the umbilicus on the ventral midline, insufflation of the abdomen, and insertion of the laparoscope through this cannula, allowing visualization of the bladder position within the abdominal cavity. A second trocar cannula is inserted on the midline just cranial to the prepuce in male dogs or directly ventral to the cranial margin of the bladder as determined by visual inspection in female dogs and male and female cats. A laparoscopic Babcock forceps is inserted through this second, more caudally located cannula to grasp the cranioventral region of the urinary bladder, near or at the bladder apex. After lengthening of the trocar incision, the trocar through which the laparoscopic Babcock forceps is passed may be removed, and the urinary bladder lifted to the prior trocar site. Traction (stay) sutures may then be placed around the intended cystotomy site, the bladder held tightly against the abdominal opening to minimize urine contamination of the peritoneal cavity, and a small full-thickness incision into the bladder allows placement of the 5-mm laparoscope or small 2.7-mm cystoscope with a 30° viewing angle. In female dogs, use of the smaller cystoscope may be used to pass from the bladder for inspection of the entire urethra and into the vestibule. In male dogs, the technique of LA cystoscopy may be modified by using a 2.5-mm flexible scope to examine the urethra to the area of the os penis.[9] If a 5-mm laparoscope is used, it may not be possible to inspect the entire urethra even in female dogs, and if visual inspection is not possible, antegrade and retrograde catheterization with copious flushing of the urethra is recommended in both males and females to ensure that no obstructive calculi, blood clots, grit, or tissue are left within the urethral lumen. Once completed, the bladder incisions may be reconstructed according to the preferences of the operating surgeon similar to an open cystotomy, using an interrupted or continuous pattern, and in a single-layer or 2-layer technique. Monofilament absorbable suture is recommended. After closure of the bladder incisions, the bladder may be returned to the abdomen, any residual CO_2 evacuated from the peritoneal cavity, and the laparoscopic trocar incisions closed according to the preferences of the operating surgeon.

Technique/Procedures

Urinary calculus removal

Two similar techniques for LA urolith removal in small animals have been described. The original technique[9] for LA cystotomy in which one of the ports is placed in a paramedian position in male dogs may be modified to allow all ports to be placed on the ventral midline.[10] Other described modifications of the original technique included a temporary cystopexy to the abdominal wall, use of a laparoscope instead of a rigid cystoscope, and retrograde pressurized flow of saline in the bladder via a Foley urinary catheter.[10] In the modified technique, once the bladder is grasped with the laparoscopic Babcock forceps, the instrument cannula is removed and the approach through the body wall on the midline is enlarged to approximately 3 to 4 cm.[10] A 360° temporary cystopexy is performed with full-thickness bites through the body wall and the bladder wall, creating a tight seal to prevent loss of urine or calculi into the peritoneal cavity.[10] Entry into the bladder lumen is made with a small stab incision, and the 6-mm laparoscopic cannula is placed through this stab incision, allowing the laparoscope to be introduced into the bladder lumen. Uroliths may then be flushed from the urinary bladder under high pressure and removed with suction attached to the ingress/egress portal of the cannula.[10] With this method, it is important to place the largest-diameter urinary catheter possible to create good retrograde flow of saline for adequate bladder inflation and visualization, and this may be a limitation in male cats because of their small urethral diameter.[10] If a rigid cystoscope is used, saline infusion may be performed through the cystoscope channel; however, this may create a forward flow of saline that may push uroliths into the urethra, and before completing the procedure, retrograde catheterization and careful flushing of the urethra are important. For uroliths too large to be removed by flushing or withdrawal through the portal in this manner, grasping forceps or basket catheters may be introduced into the urinary bladder immediately adjacent to the laparoscope. Bladder wall and body wall incisions are closed according to the preference of the operating surgeon as described earlier.

Urinary bladder polypectomy

Removal of inflammatory polyps in the urinary bladder of dogs with chronic/recurrent urinary tract infections is recommended to help manage infection and inflammation. Unlike urinary bladder neoplasia, resection with only minimal surgical margins is needed, and a technique of polypectomy via LA cystoscopy has been described.[11] Although minimizing urine contamination of the abdomen, the LA technique provided clear surgical margins and a thorough examination of the inside of the bladder.[11] The approach was made as described earlier, and the abdominal incision was enlarged sufficiently to allow exteriorization of the portion of the bladder containing the polyp. The bladder was distended with fluid, the margins of the polyp were determined through visual inspection through the scope, and a scalpel was used to incise the bladder at the margins of the polyp.[11] Bladder wall reconstruction was performed as for a standard cystotomy.

Cystopexy

Although traditionally a celiotomy has been required for cystopexy procedures in female dogs with pelvic bladder or retroflexion of the urinary bladder in perineal hernia, an LA incisional cystopexy technique has been described in dogs.[12] The patient should be placed in dorsal recumbency, clipped and aseptically prepared, and placed in a mild Trendelenburg position. A 2-portal technique may be used, with a 5-mm or 10-mm camera portal placed on the midline, just caudal to the umbilicus, and CO_2 pneumoperitoneum established according to the preference of the operating surgeon. After inspection of the caudal peritoneal cavity, a second (10-mm) portal should be placed lateral of the midline, in the right rectus abdominus muscle to allow insertion of a 10-mm laparoscopic Babcock forceps. The midportion of the bladder may be grasped by the laparoscopic Babcock forceps and a 3- to 5-cm incision extended from the site of portal introduction longitudinally in the skin and right rectus abdominus muscle. The bladder may be exteriorized. Two temporary traction sutures may be placed 3 to 5 cm apart to minimize the risk of dropping the bladder back into the peritoneal cavity, and an incisional cystopexy performed by making a 2.5- to 4-cm-long incision in a craniocaudal direction in the seromuscular layer of the bladder wall. Full-thickness incision through the bladder wall should be avoided. Similar to an incisional gastropexy, parallel continuous suture patterns of 3-0 polydioxanone may be used to appose the seromuscular layer of the bladder to the aponeurosis of the external and internal abdominal oblique muscles. The abdominal musculature and skin at the cystopexy site and camera portal site may be reconstructed with suture and pattern according to the preferences of the operating surgeon. Cystopexy performed in this manner resulted in strong adhesion between the urinary bladder and abdominal wall, with cystopexy length of 2 to 3 cm, and was a durable and acceptable alternative to a cystopexy performed through a laparotomy.[12]

Tube cystostomy

An LA approach can be useful for minimally invasive tube cystostomy in cases that require temporary or permanent diversion of urine from the urinary bladder, but in which urethral catheterization is not desired or feasible. A technique of intracorporeal laparoscopic tube cystostomy[13] has been published, and is easily adaptable to an LA technique. The patient should be positioned in dorsal recumbency, widely clipped, aseptically prepared, and placed in a mild Trendelenburg position. It may be helpful to choose an optimal cystostomy tube exit site from the body wall while the patient is awake and standing and mark this before surgery. A 2-portal technique may be used, with a 5-mm or 10-mm camera portal placed on the midline, just caudal to the umbilicus, and CO_2 pneumoperitoneum established according to the preference of the operating surgeon. The relative position of the bladder may be assessed, and the craniocaudal position of the second portal should be chosen to allow the bladder to be comfortably brought to the body wall. The second portal should be placed 5 to 10 cm to the right of the midline, at the lateral aspect of the right rectus abdominus muscle, or where preoperatively determined to be an optimal lateral position. A 10-mm portal at this site is recommended, to allow introduction of 10-mm laparoscopic Babcock forceps for the purposes of grasping and exteriorizing the bladder wall. Once the Babcock forceps has been introduced, the bladder wall grasped, and appropriate positioning confirmed, the skin and body wall incision should be extended longitudinally 4 to 6 cm from the portal (in a cranial-caudal direction), to allow the bladder to be exteriorized through the body wall. Traction sutures should be placed in the bladder to ensure that it does not retract too far back into the peritoneal cavity and a purse string suture of absorbable suture material placed in the bladder wall. With a scalpel blade, a stab incision should be made into the bladder wall of sufficient length to allow introduction of an 8- to 10-French Foley catheter. The purse string suture may be tightened and tied around the catheter, and the balloon of the Foley catheter inflated with sterile saline at the volume recommended by the manufacturer. Traction sutures may be removed, and a cystopexy may be created by suturing the seromuscular layer of the bladder to the body wall with 4 interrupted absorbable sutures placed at each of the 4 quadrants, approximately 1 cm from the entrance of the Foley catheter into the bladder. The urinary bladder may be distended by injecting sterile saline through the Foley catheter to check for patency and leakage. The muscular body wall should be reconstructed around the Foley catheter, the catheter exited through the skin, and secured to the skin by a finger trap suture. The Foley catheter should be attached to a closed urine collection system. An Elizabethan collar should be placed at all times to prevent the patient from removing the Foley catheter.

Cystostomy tubes should remain in place for at least 14 days before removal to ensure an adequate adhesion between the bladder and body wall and to reduce the possibility of urine leakage or peritonitis.[14]

LAPAROSCOPIC-ASSISTED PROCEDURES OF THE FEMALE REPRODUCTIVE TRACT

The most commonly performed LA procedure of the canine and feline female reproductive tracts is ovariohysterectomy, whether performed as an elective procedure[5,15] or as treatment of pyometra.[16] In general, the ovarian vascular pedicle is sectioned intracorporeally in these procedures, and the uterine body is ligated and sectioned extracorporeally. Two-portal and 3-portal approaches have been described for this procedure, as well as numerous variations on techniques of ovarian vascular pedicle hemostasis.[5,7,15] In 1 study of LA ovariohysterectomy, extracorporeal modified Roeder knot application, laparoscopic metal clip application, or use of a bipolar vessel-sealing device were compared for hemostasis of the ovarian pedicle, and although differences in operating time between groups were found, all methods of hemostasis were deemed safe for pedicle sectioning.[5] When performed as treatment of pyometra, LA ovariohysterectomy is a viable alternative to open celiotomy, and both 3-portal and 4-portal techniques have been described.[16,17] However intra-abdominal uterine rupture has been reported in 1 dog undergoing LA ovariohysterectomy for pyometra, requiring conversion to an open celiotomy, so careful case selection is important to maximize success and minimize risk of conversion to an open approach.[16] It has been recommended to use the LA ovariohysterectomy technique for canine pyometra in dogs weighing less than 10 kg when the uterine horn diameter is modestly sized (<2 cm) and in larger dogs when the uterine horn diameter is 4 cm or less.[16]

Patient Preparation and Positioning

Once anesthetized, the patient is placed in dorsal recumbency. Although not always necessary, a mild Trendelenburg position may minimize encroachment by cranial abdominal viscera. A tilt-table to roll the patient 15° to 20° laterally from straight dorsal recumbency to allow organs to fall toward the surgeon and better expose the ovarian pedicle can be helpful but is not a requirement. If a 2-portal technique is elected, abdominal preparation and draping need to be performed particularly widely to allow temporary sterile percutaneous access to the ovaries. In general, the operating surgeon stands on both the left and the right sides of the patient during this procedure for approach of the contralateral ovary. When the right ovary is approached, the surgeon stands on the left side of the patient and tilts the table toward the patient's left. When the left ovary is approached, the surgeon stands on the right side of the patient and tilts the table toward the patient's right. The laparoscopic tower should be placed toward the front of the patient so that the screen may be more easily shifted when the surgeon changes sides.

Approach

Original reports of LA ovariohysterectomy have described either a 2-portal or a 3-portal midline approach.[5,15] Single-portal laparoscopic ovariectomy has been reported in the veterinary literature[18,19] and may be a viable option for LA ovariohysterectomy as well with caudal placement of the operating portal to allow subsequent extracorporeal access to the uterine body, although experience with single-portal LA ovariohysterectomy has not been formally described. Establishment of pneumoperitoneum and initial portal placement are obtained according to the preference of the operating surgeon. Whether a 2-portal or 3-portal technique is elected, the placement of the first portal is usually performed 1 to 3 cm caudal to the umbilicus. After visual inspection of the abdomen, the additional portals are placed. In a 2-portal technique, the location of the second (caudal) port is chosen to facilitate access to the uterine body when the length of this incision is enlarged. In a 3-portal technique, the initial (camera portal) is placed 1 to 3 cm caudal to the umbilicus and the instrument portals are established under direct observation 3 to 5 cm cranial to the umbilicus and 3 to 5 cm cranial to the pubis. Portal sizes of either 6 mm or 11 mm are chosen based on the type of instruments that the operating surgeon wishes to use.

Technique/Procedure

Ovariohysterectomy

Using rotation provided by the table tilt and manipulation of the intestines and spleen with a blunt probe, the ovary may be visualized. For a 3-port LA ovariohysterectomy technique, the ovary is grasped with a laparoscopic Kelly forceps or a laparoscopic Babcock forceps and elevated (**Fig. 1**A). Pedicle hemostasis and sectioning are then performed according to the technique of choice; the author prefers combined coagulation and sectioning with a vessel-sealing device such as the 5-mm Ligasure Dolphin or 10-mm Ligasure Atlas handpieces (Covidien, Minneapolis, MN, USA). The procedure is repeated on the opposite ovarian pedicle, and once completed, the caudal portal approach through the skin and body wall is enlarged sufficiently that the ovaries, uterine horns, and body may be exteriorized (**Fig. 1**B). Mesometrial attachments are torn, coagulated, or ligated, and ligation and transection of the uterine body cranial to the cervix are performed in a conventional manner with absorbable monofilament suture material according to the preferences of the operating surgeon. The uterus and ovaries are removed, and the body wall incisions are repaired in the standard fashion with monofilament absorbable suture.

This technique may be modified to a 2-portal technique if desired by placing a camera port in the subumbilical position and an instrument port 3 to 5 cm cranial to the pubis. The camera is introduced through the cranial portal and a laparoscopic Kelly forceps or a laparoscopic Babcock forceps is introduced through the caudal portal. The ovary is grasped and elevated toward the ventrolateral body wall. A

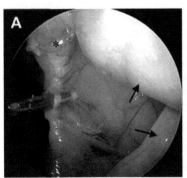
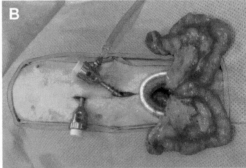

Fig. 1. LA ovariohysterectomy. (*A*) A three-port technique was used in this case of pyometra, allowing intracorporeal manipulation of the ovarian pedicles during dissection. The left ovary (*), uterine horn (*black arrows*), and vessel-sealing device can be seen coagulating/sectioning the ovarian pedicle. (*B*) After sectioning mesometrial attachments with the vessel-sealing device, the caudal portal incision was elongated, a 4-cm Alexis wound retractor placed, and the entire reproductive tract exteriorized for uterine body ligation and transection just cranial to the cervix.

transabdominal suspension suture on a large taper needle is advanced through the skin and body wall, directed around ovarian tissue, and back through the body wall. To suspend and facilitate exposure of the ovarian pedicle, the suture is pulled tight and temporarily secured by grasping both ends of the suture with mosquito hemostatic clamps at the point at which the suture ends exit the skin. The laparoscopic grasping forceps may then be withdrawn and a vessel-sealing device introduced through the free portal for coagulation and sectioning of the ovarian pedicle. If the angle of approach is not optimal with the camera introduced through the cranial portal, the surgeon may consider switching instruments between portals. Although any portion of the ovary, proper ligament, or cranial uterine horn may be used to suspend the pedicle, the author has personally found that dissection and sectioning are facilitated if more cranial placement of the suspension suture around the ovary is performed rather than caudally encompassing the proper ligament or uterus. The process is repeated on the opposite ovarian pedicle, and then both suspension sutures are released, the incision encompassing the caudal portal is extended, and the ovaries, uterine horns, and uterine body are exteriorized and removed as described earlier.

LAPAROSCOPIC-ASSISTED PROCEDURES OF THE MALE REPRODUCTIVE TRACT
Cryptorchidectomy

LA cryptorchidectomy has been described in dogs and cats and is a viable technique for identification and retrieval of abdominally retained testicles.[20,21] In veterinary patients, castration is the recommended treatment of cryptorchidism, because the incidence of testicular neoplasia in abdominally retained testicles is nearly 14 times higher than in descended testicles.[22] An LA approach to retained testicles allows accurate localization and visual confirmation of anatomic structures and still provides the advantages of a minimally invasive technique. Minilaparotomies and use of a spay hook without laparoscopic visualization to castrate cryptorchid animals have been reported; however, without appropriate visualization, unacceptable complications including urethral avulsion, inadvertent prostatectomy, and ureteral/urethral trauma have been described.[20] LA procedures minimize risks of inaccurate structure identification and iatrogenic tissue damage, maximize patient recovery, and minimize the need for specialized equipment or techniques such as intracorporeal suturing, laparoscopic clip appliers, or vessel-sealing devices for fully intracorporeal procedures. Accurate identification of the location of the retained testicle (inguinal vs abdominal) is useful preoperative information, and abdominal ultrasonography to confirm testicle location is recommended before surgery. However, if ultrasonography is unavailable, insertion of the laparoscope through a single portal allows visual confirmation of the testicle location by evaluating the presence or absence of the ductus deferens and testicular vessels exiting the abdomen via the inguinal ring. If these structures are observed exiting the inguinal rings bilaterally, then, the abdominal procedure is aborted, and exploration for the nondescended testicle(s) can be limited to the subcutaneous space of the inguinal region.

Patient preparation and positioning
Once anesthetized, the patient is placed in dorsal recumbency. Although not always necessary, a mild Trendelenburg position may minimize encroachment by cranial abdominal viscera.

Approach
Pneumoperitoneum may be established either by Veress needle placement or the open (Hasson) technique according to the preferences of the operating surgeon,

with the abdomen insufflated to an intra-abdominal pressure of 8 to 12 mm Hg. The general technique for LA cryptorchidectomy for these procedures includes insertion of a 6-mm trocar cannula at the level of, or just slightly caudal to, the umbilicus on the ventral midline, insufflation of the abdomen, and insertion of the laparoscope through this cannula, allowing visualization of the caudal abdominal cavity. The abdomen is explored beginning with visual inspection of the inguinal rings to confirm that the testicle(s) have truly not exited the peritoneal cavity.

Technique/procedure

The original technique described placement of a second 6-mm portal ventral and lateral to the identified cryptorchid testicle, grasping the identified testicle with laparoscopic forceps, and enlarging the trocar site for withdrawal of the testicle outside the abdominal cavity.[20] Alternatively, if the retained testicle seems mobile, the second 6-mm trocar cannula may be inserted 3 to 4 cm caudal to the first on the midline (cranial to the prepuce in male dogs or midway between the first portal and the pubis in male cats) for introduction of a laparoscopic grasping forceps. The abdominal testicle(s) may then be brought toward the midline, the incision enlarged to connect the 2 portal sites, and the testicle exteriorized for extracorporeal ligation and transection of the vascular supply and ductus deferens. Once excised, the linea alba, subcutaneous tissue, and skin may be closed in the standard fashion, according to the preferences of the operating surgeon. If the testicle cannot be mobilized and exteriorized on the midline, then a paramedian second portal placement and testicle exteriorization may be performed as originally described.[20,21]

LAPAROSCOPIC-ASSISTED PROCEDURES OF THE GASTROINTESTINAL TRACT

Common procedures of the gastrointestinal tract in veterinary medicine that lend themselves to an LA approach include LA gastropexy, LA small intestinal biopsy or resection/anastomosis, LA colopexy, LA pancreatic biopsy, and LA enterostomy tube placement. Procedures like pancreatic biopsy are commonly performed intracorporeally using laparoscopic cup biopsy forceps. In a study of laparoscopic pancreatic biopsy in cats, the laparoscopic punch cup forceps provided high-quality pancreatic biopsy samples with an average size of 5 mm × 4 mm on two-dimensional cut section.[23] However, if a larger sample is desired, the right limb of the pancreas may be exteriorized in an LA approach for sampling.[24] A recent study[25] evaluated different access incision locations on the ventral abdominal midline for minimally invasive access and collection of multiple organ biopsy samples in cats. A 3-cm access incision centered midway between the caudal margin of the xiphoid cartilage and the umbilicus was found to provide access for minimally invasive biopsy of most organs in this population of cats, including liver, pancreas, stomach, small intestine, and mesenteric lymph nodes, although access to all hepatic lobes and all parts of the pancreas was inconsistent.[25] Because of this finding, when considering minimally invasive extracorporeal organ biopsy, thorough preoperative evaluation is important to rule out concurrent disease, laparoscopic visual inspection should be combined with exteriorization of the organs of interest, and the operating surgeon should be confident that no important pathologic changes are missed.[25] Visceral organ mobility is more limited in dogs than in cats, and in dogs, the Alexis wound retractor position should be chosen based on laparoscopic confirmation of the location of the primary organ(s) of interest.

Because pneumoperitoneum is lost when the incision is extended and the visceral structures of interest are exteriorized, it is recommended to perform these types of biopsies at the end of a laparoscopic procedure that might also include intracorporeal solid parenchymal organ biopsies. After visual inspection and any desired intracorporeal parenchymal organ biopsies, the telescope can be removed, and the port incision enlarged to allow the placement of an Alexis wound retractor. This device applies circumferential force at the wound margin, converting a linear incision to a circular orifice, which minimizes compression of the mesenteric root and subsequent vascular compromise that may be associated with exteriorization of viscera through a nonretracted body wall incision. It also allows for improved exteriorization of bowel and mesenteric lymph nodes and prevents contamination of the wound margins, which has been shown in human studies to reduce wound infection rates.[26–28]

Patient Preparation and Positioning

Once anesthetized, the patient is placed in dorsal recumbency. If an LA gastropexy procedure is to be performed, dogs should be clipped more laterally along the right cranial abdomen to facilitate the paramedian trocar placement and approach in this region. The laparoscopic tower should be placed toward the front of the patient slightly across the table from the operating surgeon, depending on the procedure(s) elected.

Approach

Laparoscopic portal placement depends on the procedure being performed. In general, a camera portal is placed on the ventral midline in the subumbilical region; however, the location of the remainder of the portals placed depends on the procedure(s) to be performed.

Technique/Procedures

Laparoscopic-assisted gastropexy

The efficacy of incisional gastropexy for the long-term prevention of gastric dilation-volvulus in dogs has been confirmed, and several minimally invasive techniques of laparoscopic and LA incisional gastropexy have been described.[29,30] LA gastropexy has been shown to be quick, technically simple, safe, and effective in forming a strong fibrous adhesion between the stomach and body wall that provides effective prevention of gastric volvulus.[31,32] The patient is positioned in dorsal recumbency, and a camera portal is placed in the subumbilical region and the peritoneal cavity insufflated. Under visualization through the laparoscope, an 11-mm trocar cannula is placed lateral to the right margin of the rectus abdominus muscle, caudal to the margin of the last rib, enabling passage of a 10-mm laparoscopic Babcock forceps. The pyloric antrum approximately 5 to 7 cm orad to the pylorus is grasped using the Babcock forceps, the incision associated with the lateral portal is enlarged, and the cannula and Babcock forceps are withdrawn together from the abdomen, evacuating the pneumoperitoneum and allowing the pyloric antrum to be exteriorized.[31] Care should be taken to ensure that the pyloric antrum is not twisted or kinked into an abnormal position that could affect gastric outflow. Temporary traction sutures are then placed approximately 4 to 5 cm apart in the pyloric antrum, defining the extent of the anticipated gastropexy incision site in the stomach wall. Avoiding the blood vessels arising from the greater and lesser curvatures of the stomach, a longitudinal seromuscular incision is made into the pyloric antrum, in the same manner as an open incisional gastropexy procedure, with care not to penetrate the mucosa/submucosal layer. The edges of the seromuscular incision are sutured to the edges of the transversus abdominus muscle incision with 2 parallel continuous sutures with 2-0 polydioxanone. The gastropexy site may be visually inspected using the laparoscope placed through the midline portal to ensure appropriate positioning before closure. The oblique muscle layers, subcutaneous layer, and skin are subsequently closed routinely over the gastropexy site, and the portal site on the midline is closed in the standard manner. Modifications to this technique, including techniques for combined ovariectomy and LA gastropexy, have been described.[33,34]

Laparoscopic-assisted small intestinal biopsy or resection/anastomosis

LA intestinal biopsy and intestinal resection and anastomosis are an effective method for diagnostic investigation of chronic disease as well as for resection of modestly sized discrete intestinal masses and may be performed with single-portal, 2 ventral midline portal, or 3 ventral midline portal laparoscopic techniques.[24,25,35,36] After laparoscopic abdominal exploration, longitudinal enlargement of 1 of the abdominal portal incisions on the ventral midline is performed to create a 3-cm to 4-cm celiotomy incision, and an Alexis wound retractor is placed. The portal chosen is based on the location of the intestinal lesion: use of a portal near the umbilicus was used for duodenal and jejunal lesions and a more caudal portal for ileal, cecal, or colonic lesions in a small case series of dogs and cats.[35] The intestine is exteriorized systematically until the desired segment is identified, and surgical biopsy or resection/anastomosis is performed while the bowel is exteriorized. Incisional biopsy of mesenteric lymph nodes at the root of the mesentery may also be performed at this time. Copious local lavage is performed before replacing the bowel segment into the abdomen, the wound retractor is removed, and the small celiotomy is closed in the standard fashion.

Laparoscopic-assisted enterostomy tube placement

LA enterostomy tube placement has been described by several investigators.[37–39] In the original technique described by Rawlings and colleagues,[37] the first (camera) portal is inserted on the ventral midline just caudal to the umbilicus, and after establishment of pneumoperitoneum, a second portal is placed lateral to the right rectus abdominus muscle. A laparoscopic Babcock forceps introduced through the lateral portal is used to grasp the duodenum and elevate it to the incision made for the cannula. The cannula is withdrawn, and the antimesenteric surface of the duodenum is sutured to the abdominal wall. A purse string suture is placed in the antimesenteric aspect of the jejunum, a stab incision is made in the center of the purse string suture, and a feeding tube is inserted through the purse string into the small intestinal lumen. The purse string is tightened around the feeding tube and tied, the tube is well secured, and the incision is closed. This technique was modified by Hewitt and colleagues,[38] and animals in this study were positioned in right lateral recumbency. This technique has also subsequently been reported to have been performed using lift laparoscopy instead of pneumoperitoneum to generate working space within the abdomen.[39]

Laparoscopic-assisted colopexy

Techniques for LA incisional colopexy have been reported in a case report of a single cat[40] and a small case series of dogs.[41] Permanent adhesions were created between the descending colon and body wall, using an LA extracorporeally sutured technique. Animals were positioned in dorsal recumbency and a 2-portal or 3-portal technique was used. For the 2-portal technique, the camera portal was placed on the ventral midline, and the second portal placed in the left inguinal region.[40] The descending colon was grasped with forceps placed through the lateral portal and the incision enlarged to allow exteriorization of the colon.[40] A seromuscular incision was made in the colon on the antimesenteric surface and the seromuscular layer of the colon was apposed to the body wall, similar to the manner of an LA gastropexy.[40]

LAPAROSCOPIC-ASSISTED SPLENECTOMY

Although several reports in the veterinary literature have documented laparoscopic splenectomy,[42–45] description of LA splenectomy is less common. Recently, LA splenectomy in conjunction with LA intestinal biopsy was reported in a cat, performed through an access incision centered over the umbilicus.[46] With the advent of larger wound retraction systems as described earlier, there is no reason that LA splenectomy should not become more common (**Fig. 2**). Dogs undergoing laparoscopic splenectomy showed fewer signs of pain, had fewer wound complications, and experienced less blood loss than those undergoing open surgery, although the laparoscopic technique did require longer surgical time compared with open splenectomy.[42]

Patient Preparation and Positioning

Once anesthetized the patient is placed in dorsal recumbency. In general, the operating surgeon stands on the right side of the patient. The laparoscopic tower should be placed directly across from the operating surgeon or toward the front of the patient.

Approach

The technique is similar for other LA procedures. A camera portal is typically placed on the ventral midline in the subumbilical region and a second portal is placed on the ventral midline cranial or caudal to the camera portal, depending on whether other procedures will be performed in addition. After visual inspection of the abdomen is performed, in which the size and position of the spleen are assessed, and other parenchymal organ biopsies are performed if needed (eg, liver biopsy), one of the

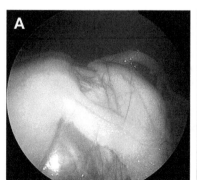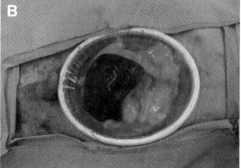

Fig. 2. LA splenectomy. (*A*) Ventral midline portals were initially placed and a laparoscope introduced for visual inspection of the liver and other viscera, and confirmation of splenic position for wound retractor placement. Here, position of the splenic mass can be seen through the laparoscope, allowing the surgeon to fine-tune incision enlargement for optimal LA exposure. (*B*) The portals were subsequently removed, the incision elongated, and the 10-cm Alexis wound retractor placed. Splenectomy was performed using a vessel-sealing device for coagulation/sectioning along the vascular hilus.

portal sites can be extended, and an appropriately sized Alexis wound retractor is placed.

Technique/Procedure

Vascular dissection along the hilus of the spleen may be initiated at the tail of the spleen and progress toward the head of the spleen. Hemostasis and transection along the hilus are most easily achieved using a vessel-sealing device; however, standard suture ligation may also be performed. Gentle digital traction can be used to retract the spleen out of the portal incision as dissection progresses and the hilar vessels are ligated and transected. Care should be taken not to cause iatrogenic damage to the pancreas, or hemorrhage from overzealous retraction.[46] If tension is judged to be excessive during digital retraction, the telescope can be placed through the Alexis device, with simultaneous elevation of the body wall to allow visualization of the area of the head of the spleen.[46] The portal or miniceliotomy sites may be closed in a routine manner.

COMPLICATIONS AND MANAGEMENT

General complications of LA procedures can include:

- Access injury to viscera (eg, splenic laceration) from portal or Veress needle placement
- Hemorrhage from solid-organ biopsy sites
- Seroma formation at port sites if dead space is not eliminated during closure
- Surgical site infections
- Body wall herniation of viscera through incompletely reconstructed port sites
- Port site metastasis of neoplastic lesions if the body wall is not protected during retrieval of specimens

Specific complications related to the specific organ system or type of procedure should also be considered. For example:

- Leakage from needle holes in the colon has been described associated with an LA colopexy in a patient with perineal hernia.[12]
- Technical difficulties such as chronic cystitis resulting in a severely thickened and noncompliant/poorly distensible bladder, or inadequate flow of saline obscuring visualization may necessitate conversion to an open cystotomy.
- Failure of complete urocystolith removal has been documented in 10% to 20% of small animal patients undergoing open or LA cystotomy.[10,47] Even after LA cystotomy, postoperative radiographs are recommended to make sure that no uroliths are left in the urinary system.
- Conversion to open laparotomy may be necessary during LA intestinal mass resections when the mass has adhesions to surrounding organs or the margins of the mass cannot be clearly visualized.[25]

POSTOPERATIVE CARE

Although in general, minimally invasive procedures are associated with improved postoperative comfort,[15] a more rapid return to normal activity,[48,49] and at times shorter hospital stays, individualized patient care should include:

- Appropriate postoperative analgesia (opiate analgesics or nonsteroidal antiinflammatory medications if not contraindicated)
- Postoperative cold compressing of surgical incisions

- Limited activity until suture removal (2 weeks postoperatively)
- Individualized monitoring and therapeutic recommendations, depending on the procedure performed and diagnostic results

REFERENCES

1. Robinson CN, Balentine CJ, Marshall CL, et al. Minimally invasive surgery improves short-term outcomes in elderly colorectal cancer patients. J Surg Res 2011;166:182–8.
2. Lansdowne JL, Mehler SJ, Boure LB. Minimally invasive abdominal and thoracic surgery: principles and instrumentation. Compend Contin Educ Vet 2012;34:E1–9.
3. Monnet E, Twedt DC. Laparoscopy. Vet Clin North Am Small Anim Pract 2003;33: 1147–63.
4. Robertson E, Webb C, Twedt D. Diagnostic laparoscopy in the cat 1. Common procedures. J Feline Med Surg 2014;16:5–16.
5. Mayhew PD, Brown DC. Comparison of three techniques for ovarian pedicle hemostasis during laparoscopic-assisted ovariohysterectomy. Vet Surg 2007;36:541–7.
6. Fiorbianco V, Skalicky M, Doerner, et al. Right intercostal insertion of a Veress needle for laparoscopy in dogs. Vet Surg 2012;41(3):367–73.
7. Gower S, Mayhew P. Canine laparoscopic and laparoscopic-assisted ovariohysterectomy and ovariectomy. Compend Contin Educ Vet 2008;30(8):430–2, 433, 436, 438, 440. Available at: http://www.ncbi.nlm.nih.gov/pubmed/18833541.
8. Arulpragasam SP, Case JB, Ellison GW. Evaluation of costs and time required for laparoscopic-assisted versus open cystotomy for urinary cystolith removal in dogs: 43 cases (2009-2012). J Am Vet Med Assoc 2013;243:703–8.
9. Rawlings CA, Mahaffey MB, Barsanti JA, et al. Use of laparoscopic-assisted cystoscopy for removal of urinary calculi in dogs. J Am Vet Med Assoc 2003; 222(6):759–61. Available at: http://www.ncbi.nlm.nih.gov/pubmed/12675298.
10. Pinel CB, Monnet E, Reems MR. Laparoscopic-assisted cystotomy for urolith removal in dogs and cats–23 cases. Can Vet J 2013;54(1):36–41.
11. Rawlings CA. Resection of inflammatory polyps in dogs using laparoscopic-assisted cystopexy. J Am Anim Hosp Assoc 2007;43(6):342–6. Available at: http://www.ncbi.nlm.nih.gov/pubmed/17975217.
12. Rawlings CA, Howerth EW, Mahaffey MB, et al. Laparoscopic-assisted cystopexy in dogs. Am J Vet Res 2002;63(9):1226–31. Available at: http://www.ncbi.nlm.nih. gov/pubmed/12224851.
13. Zhang JT, Wang HB, Shi J, et al. Laparoscopy for percutaneous tube cystostomy placement in dogs. J Am Vet Med Assoc 2010;236(9):975–7. Available at: http:// www.ncbi.nlm.nih.gov/pubmed/20433397.
14. Hayashi K, Hardie RJ. Use of cystostomy tubes in small animals. Compend Contin Educ Vet 2003;25(12):928–35.
15. Devitt CM, Cox RE, Hailey JJ. Duration, complications, stress, and pain of open ovariohysterectomy versus a simple method of laparoscopic-assisted ovariohysterectomy in dogs. J Am Vet Med Assoc 2005;227(6):921–7. Available at: http:// www.ncbi.nlm.nih.gov/pubmed/16190590.
16. Adamovich-Rippe KN, Mayhew PD, Runge JJ, et al. Evaluation of laparoscopic-assisted ovariohysterectomy for treatment of canine pyometra. Vet Surg 2013;42: 572–8.
17. Minami S, Okamoto Y, Eguchi H, et al. Successful laparoscopy assisted ovariohysterectomy in two dogs with pyometra. J Vet Med Sci 1997;59:845–7.

18. Dupre G, Fiorbianco V, Skalicky M, et al. Laparoscopic ovariectomy in dogs, comparison between single portal and two-portal access. Vet Surg 2009;38(7): 818–24.

19. Manassero M, Leperlier D, Vallefuoco R, et al. Laparoscopic ovariectomy in dogs using a single-port multiple-access device. Vet Rec 2012;171(3):69.

20. Miller NA, Van Lue SJ, Rawlings CA. Use of laparoscopic assisted cryptorchidectomy in dogs and cats. J Am Vet Med Assoc 2004;224(6):875–8. Available at: http://www.ncbi.nlm.nih.gov/pubmed/15070057.

21. Mayhew P. Laparoscopic and laparoscopic-assisted cryptorchidectomy in dogs and cats. Compend Contin Educ Vet 2009;31(6):E9. Available at: http://www.ncbi.nlm.nih.gov/pubmed/19746347.

22. Hayes HM, Pendergrass TW. Canine testicular tumors: epidemiologic features of 410 dogs. Int J Cancer 1976;18:482–7.

23. Cosford KL, Shmon CL, Myers SL, et al. Prospective evaluation of laparoscopic pancreatic biopsies in 11 healthy cats. J Vet Intern Med 2010;24(1):104–13. Available at: http://www.ncbi.nlm.nih.gov/pubmed/19925571.

24. Mayhew P. Surgical views: techniques for laparoscopic and laparoscopic-assisted biopsy of abdominal organs. Compend Contin Educ Vet 2009;31(4): 170–6. Available at: http://www.ncbi.nlm.nih.gov/pubmed/19517409.

25. Mayhew PD, Mayhew KN, Shilo-Benjamini Y, et al. Prospective evaluation of access incision position for minimally invasive surgical organ exposure in cats. J Am Vet Med Assoc 2014;245:1129–34.

26. Horiuchi T, Tanishima H, Tamagawa K, et al. Randomized controlled investigation of the anti-infective properties of the Alexis retractor/protector of incision sites. J Trauma 2007;62:212–5.

27. Cheng KP, Roslani AC, Sehha N, et al. ALEXIS O-Ring wound retractor vs conventional wound protection for the prevention of surgical site infections in colorectal resections. Colorectal Dis 2012;14:e346–51.

28. Robertson E, Webb C, Twedt D. Diagnostic laparoscopy in the cat 2. Common procedures. J Feline Med Surg 2014;16:18–26.

29. Benitez ME, Schmiedt CW, Radlinsky MG, et al. Efficacy of incisional gastropexy for prevention of GDV in dogs. J AM Anim Hosp Assoc 2013;9(3):185–9. Available at: http://www.ncbi.nlm.nih.gov/pubmed/23535748.

30. Runge JJ, Mayhew P, Rawlings CA. Laparoscopic-assisted and laparoscopic prophylactic gastropexy: indications and techniques. Compend Contin Educ Vet 2009;31(2):E2. Available at: http://www.ncbi.nlm.nih.gov/pubmed/19288436.

31. Rawlings CA, Foutz TL, Mahaffey MB, et al. A rapid and strong laparoscopic-assisted gastropexy in dogs. Am J Vet Res 2001;62(6):871–5. Available at: http://www.ncbi.nlm.nih.gov/pubmed/11400843.

32. Rawlings CA, Mahaffey MB, Bement S, et al. Prospective evaluation of laparoscopic-assisted gastropexy in dogs susceptible to gastric dilatation. J Am Vet Med Assoc 2002;221(11):1576–81. Available at: http://www.ncbi.nlm.nih.gov/pubmed/12479327.

33. Runge JJ, Mayhew PD. Evaluation of single port access gastropexy and ovariectomy using articulating instruments and angled telescopes in dogs. Vet Surg 2013;42:807–13.

34. Rivier P, Furneaux R, Viguier E. Combined laparoscopic ovariectomy and laparoscopic-assisted gastropexy in dogs susceptible to gastric dilatation-volvulus. Can Vet J 2011;52:62–6.

35. Gower SB, Mayhew PD. A wound retraction device for laparoscopic-assisted intestinal surgery in dogs and cats. Vet Surg 2011;40:485–9.
36. Case BJ, Ellison G. Single incision laparoscopic-assisted intestinal surgery (SILAIS) in 7 dogs and 1 cat. Vet Surg 2013;42:629–34.
37. Rawlings CA, Howerth EW, Bement S, et al. Laparoscopic-assisted enterostomy tube placement and full-thickness biopsy of the jejunum with serosal patching in dogs. Am J Vet Res 2002;63(9):1313–9. Available at: http://www.ncbi.nlm.nih.gov/pubmed/12224867.
38. Hewitt SA, Brisson BA, Sinclair MD, et al. Evaluation of laparoscopic-assisted placement of jejunostomy feeding tubes in dogs. J Am Vet Med Assoc 2004;225(1):65–71. Available at: http://www.ncbi.nlm.nih.gov/pubmed/15239475.
39. Fransson BA, Ragel CA. Lift laparoscopy in dogs and cats: 12 cases (2008-2009). J Am Vet Med Assoc 2011;239:1574–9.
40. Secchi P, Castagnino Kunert Filho H, Sussel Feranti JP, et al. Laparoscopic-assisted incisional colopexy by 2 portals access in a domestic cat with recurrent rectal prolapse. J Feline Med Surg 2011;14(2):169–70.
41. Mathon DH, Palierne S, Meynaud-Collard P, et al. Laparoscopic-assisted colopexy and sterilization in male dogs: short-term results and physiologic consequences. Vet Surg 2011;40:500–8.
42. Stedile R, Beck CA, Schiochet F, et al. Laparoscopic versus open splenectomy in dogs. Pesq Vet Bras 2009;29:653–60.
43. Collard F, Nadeau ME, Carmel EN. Laparoscopic splenectomy for treatment of splenic hemangiosarcoma in a dog. Vet Surg 2010;39:870–2.
44. Bakhtiari J, Tavakoli A, Khalaj A, et al. Minimally invasive total splenectomy in dogs: a clinical report. Int J Vet Res 2011;5:9–12.
45. Shaver SL, Mayhew PD, Steffey MA, et al. Short-term outcome of multiple-port laparoscopic splenectomy in 10 dogs. Vet Surg 2015;44(Suppl 1):71–5. Available at: http://www.ncbi.nlm.nih.gov/pubmed/25522804.
46. O'Donnell E, Mayhew P, Culp W, et al. Laparoscopic splenectomy: operative technique and outcome in three cats. J Feline Med Surg 2013;15:48–52.
47. Grant DC, Harper TA, Werre SR. Frequency of incomplete urolith removal, complications, and diagnostic imaging following cystotomy for removal of uroliths from the lower urinary tract in dogs: 128 cases (1994-2006). J Am Vet Med Assoc 2010;236(7):763–6.
48. Mayhew PD, Brown DC. Prospective evaluation of two intra-corporeally sutured prophylactic laparoscopic gastropexy techniques compared to laparoscopic-assisted gastropexy in dogs. Vet Surg 2009;38:738–46.
49. Culp WTN, Mayhew PD, Brown DC. The effect of laparoscopic versus open ovariectomy on postsurgical activity in small dogs. Vet Surg 2009;38:811–7.

Advances in Laparoscopic Surgery

Chloe Wormser, VMD, Jeffrey J. Runge, DVM*

KEYWORDS

- Veterinary • Laparoscopy • Canine • Feline • Single port • SILS • SPA
- Minimally invasive surgery

KEY POINTS

- In an attempt to make minimally invasive techniques even more minimal, surgeons are exploring new approaches to abdominal entry that reduce the overall number of points of entry.
- The single-port platform has shown promise as a potentially less-invasive alternative to multiport laparoscopic surgery.
- The single-port platform enables all the individual laparoscopic instruments, including the telescope, to pass through the same abdominal incision.
- There have been several published reports documenting the efficacy and safety of single-port procedures in veterinary patients in recent years.

INTRODUCTION

Over the past decade, minimally invasive surgery has gained widespread acceptance in the veterinary community, with benefits including but not limited to improved cosmesis, reduced surgical trauma and postoperative pain, and expedited patient recovery times.[1–6] With the constantly evolving stream of technological advances and instrumentation, minimally invasive surgical techniques have been continually improving, providing a higher standard of care to veterinary patients than was possible before.

SINGLE-PORT ACCESS SURGERY

In an attempt to make minimally invasive techniques even more minimal, human and veterinary surgeons have begun to explore novel approaches to abdominal entry that

The authors have nothing to disclose.

Section of Surgery, Department of Clinical Studies, University of Pennsylvania, School of Veterinary Medicine, 3900 Delancey Street, Philadelphia, PA 19104, USA

* Corresponding author.

E-mail address: jrunge@vet.upenn.edu

http://dx.doi.org/10.1016/j.cvsm.2015.08.001
0195-5616/16/$ – see front matter
vetsmall.theclinics.com

either reduce the overall number of trocar-cannula assemblies placed through the abdominal wall or eliminate them completely by using a natural orifice.[7] This has led to the development of several new minimally invasive access platforms; the most notable are single-port access surgery and natural orifice transluminal endoscopic surgery (NOTES).[7–9] To date, single-port access surgery has emerged as the most technically feasible reduced access platform for the majority of surgeons and, therefore, is the topic of discussion. NOTES is still in its infancy and has not yet been broadly implemented; therefore, it is not discussed further. NOTES, however, will likely gain more widespread acceptance in years to come as the surgical field moves toward the paradigm of truly scarless procedures.

Principles of Single-port Access Surgery

The single-port platform has shown promise as a potentially less-invasive alternative to multiport laparoscopic techniques.[10–14] The principles of single-port surgery are similar to conventional multiport laparoscopy, although inherent differences exist. These differences must be recognized and carefully considered by the surgeon prior to attempting any single-port procedure to minimize potential surgical complications and patient morbidity.

The single-port platform enables all the individual laparoscopic instruments, including the telescope, to pass through the same single abdominal incision without compromising the safety and efficacy of the procedure.[15] Having only 1 point of abdominal entry and the resulting close proximity of instruments and optics increases, however, the technical complexity of surgery due to reduced working space, inadequate triangulation, compromised field of view, decreased exposure, and frequent instrument collisions.[16] Fortunately, several concurrent technological advances in instrumentation and optics have allowed surgeons to overcome many of these technical difficulties, notably the development of angled telescopes and angled or articulating instruments.[15] These innovations have dramatically improved the ease and efficacy by which surgeons can perform single-port procedures by minimizing instrument crowding, maximizing surgeon working space, and allowing a sufficient degree of triangulation.[15,16]

Human Applications

There has been a pronounced emergence of single-port procedures for children and adults in recent years, a majority of which have been successfully adapted from common multiport laparoscopic abdominal procedures, including cholecystectomy,[17–19] adrenalectomy,[20–22] nephrectomy,[22,23] appendectomy,[24] hemicolectomy,[25] hysterectomy,[26–29] prostatectomy,[30,31] and orchidopexy.[32,33] In human patients, it has been suggested that potential advantages of single-port surgery over conventional multiport laparoscopy include superior cosmesis through a relatively hidden umbilical scar, decreased morbidity from visceral and vascular injury during trocar placement, and reduced rate of postoperative wound infection and hernia formation.[12] Comparative trials in humans, however, have yet to demonstrate significant differences between single-port and multiport laparoscopy with regard to postoperative complications, postoperative pain, duration of hospital stay, and cosmetic results.[13,14] Importantly, clinical case series and laboratory-based skill acquisition studies have identified unique surgeon requirements of single-port surgery, with skill sets and ergonomic demands that cannot be directly adapted from existing multiport laparoscopic experience.[34] Thus, additional training should be undertaken prior to attempting single-port procedures to minimize the likelihood of complications and prolonged surgical times.

Veterinary Applications

Within the field of veterinary laparoscopy, there has also been a drive toward reduced portal surgery for several common abdominal procedures. A variety of 2-port laparoscopic-assisted techniques have been described over the past 15 years, including gastropexy,[35] cystopexy,[36] cystoscopic urinary calculi removal,[37] and cryptorchidectomy.[38] Within the past 5 years, the single-port platform has emerged as a viable minimally invasive option for procedures, including the ovariectomy (OVE),[39,40] OVE in combination with gastropexy,[41] abdominal explore for foreign body retrieval or intestinal biopsy,[42,43] hepatic biopsy,[44] and cryptorchidectomy.[45] There have been several published reports documenting the efficacy and safety of single-port procedures in veterinary patients, and the learning curve for the single-port OVE has also been described.[46] Studies comparing the results of single-port access to more traditional multiport access and open surgical techniques, however, are currently lacking in the veterinary literature.

SINGLE-PORT ENTRY DEVICES

The devices used for single-port surgery can be broadly classified as (1) specifically manufactured devices for single-port laparoscopy, (2) standard instruments and trocar-cannula assemblies used for conventional laparoscopy inserted through a single skin incision, or (3) innovative adaptations of equipment not primarily intended for laparoscopy.

Insertion Techniques for Commercially Available Single-Port Devices

Devices specifically manufactured for single-port surgery are inserted through a single full-thickness abdominal incision. These devices have multiple 5-mm to 12-mm access channels that enable an array of instruments to enter the abdominal cavity.

SILS Port

A 2-cm to 3-cm minilaparotomy is created in advance for insertion of the port (**Fig. 1**). A small amount of sterile lubricant is applied to the base of the port. The port base is then clamped with 2 curved Rochester-Carmalt forceps in a staggered fashion. Varying techniques have been described for inserting the port into the abdominal

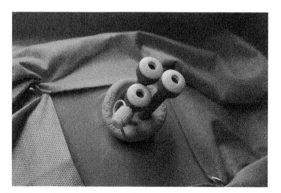

Fig. 1. SILS Port. The flexible port construction facilities easy placement, conforms to the incision to maintain pneumoperitoneum, and allows maximal maneuverability of instruments. The port can be used with three 5-mm cannulas or two 5-mm cannulas and one 10-mm or 12-mm cannula to accommodate a variety of laparoscopic instruments.

incision; it can be performed without abdominal wall countertraction or with a form of countertraction, such as grasping the facial edges with 2 large rat-toothed tissue forceps, Army-Navy retractors, or stay sutures. The tips of the Rochester-Carmalt forceps are directed into the incision in a cranial direction, toward the diaphragm and away from underlying viscera. Once the base is seated within the incision, the clamps are released to allow the port to expand and fit snugly within the incision. Three 5-mm cannulas (supplied with the port) are then inserted into the access channels with the aid of a 5-mm blunt obturator. The SILS Port (Covidien, Mansfield, Massachusetts) is also supplied with a 12-mm or 15-mm cannula to allow for use of larger instruments.

Advantages of the SILS Port include the relative ease of insertion and reinsertion during a procedure and its ability to fit snugly within the incision preventing loss of pneumoperitoneum. A study has been published within the veterinary literature evaluating the effect of standard decontamination and sterilization methods on sterility after reuse of the SILS device.[47]

EndoCone Port

A 3-cm minilaparotomy is created in advance for port insertion (**Fig. 2**). The bulkhead seal is removed, and a small amount of sterile lubricant is applied to the positive threads of the conical port. The flanged edge of the port is then inserted into the abdominal incision and threaded 360° in a clockwise direction. During port insertion, abdominal viscera are observed through the port to ensure that no bowel or omental entrapment occurs. Once the threaded cannula is in place, the EndoCone port (Karl Storz, Goleta, California) is capped by snapping the bulkhead into position.

An advantage is the EndoCone is that the bulkhead that can be removed repeatedly during the procedure without compromising the ability to reinsufflate the abdomen, thus enabling tissue removal at any time during the procedure. Another major benefit of the EndoCone is its ability to be steam sterilized in an autoclave.

GelPOINT Access System

A 2-cm to 7-cm minilaparotomy incision is created in advance for insertion of the port (**Fig. 3**). The GelPOINT access system (Applied Medical, Rancho Santa Margarita, California) consists of a wound retractor, GelSeal cap, and four 5-mm to 10-mm cannulas. The wound retractor is inserted by passing the inner flexible ring through the

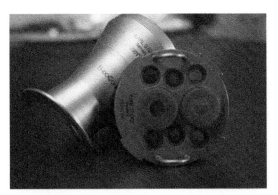

Fig. 2. EndoCone port. The EndoCone port has a bulkhead seal cap, which houses 8 valved access channels that accommodate a variety of laparoscopic instruments. Removal of the bulkhead allows for robust tissue removal during single-port laparoscopic procedures. (*Courtesy of* J. Brad Case DVM, MS, DACVS, University of Florida, Gainesville, FL, USA.)

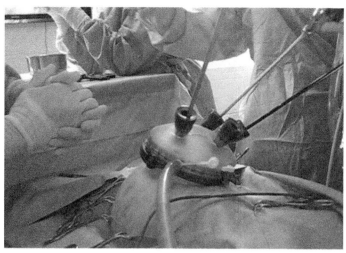

Fig. 3. GelPOINT access system. This access system is comprised of a 360° wound retractor, GelSeal cap, and multiple access sleeves.

abdominal incision. The outer ring is then rolled until it reaches the incision edge, resulting in radial wound retraction. The cannulas are inserted through the GelSeal cap, which is then fitted to the outer ring of the wound retractor.

There are several advantages to using the GelPOINT system. The wound retractor sleeve is able to accommodate the widest range of body wall thicknesses compared with other single-port devices. Additionally, the wound retractor can accommodate a 7-cm incision, which enables robust tissue removal. Lastly, the GelSeal cap can be removed and reattached repeatedly during the procedure without compromising the ability to reinsufflate the abdomen.

TriPort System

With the TriPort system (Olympus, Center Valley, Pennsylvania), a 1.5-cm to 2-cm mini-laparotomy incision is made prior to port placement (**Fig. 4**). A small amount of

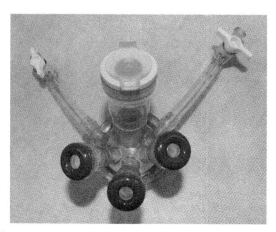

Fig. 4. TriPort system.

sterile lubricant can be applied to the inner retractor ring of the device to aid in its insertion. The device is placed into the abdominal incision by directing the internal ring of the wound retractor through the abdominal incision. The inner ring is then released from its introducer and adjusted so it sits flush against the inner body wall. The transparent sleeve attached to the inner ring is pulled up and away from the patient while the outer ring is simultaneously pushed down toward the incision. The inner and outer rings are firmly pushed together while the plastic sleeve is pulled to ensure they sit tightly against the abdominal wall. The excess transparent plastic sleeve is cut, allowing 1 cm to 2 cm of excess to be folded into the incision. The soft plastic trocar-cap is then firmly fitted onto the outer ring.

Advantages to using this device are similar to the GelPOINT system. The retractor sleeve is able to accommodate a wide range of body wall thicknesses, and the soft outer cap can be removed and reattached repeatedly during the procedure to allow tissue extraction without compromising the ability to reinsufflate the abdomen.

INSERTION TECHNIQUES FOR STANDARD TROCARS USED IN SINGLE-PORT ENTRY
Single-port Access Technique

A 1.5-cm to 2-cm skin incision is made on ventral midline in the region of the umbilicus (**Fig. 5**). Using the Hasson abdominal access technique, a 5-mm blunt laparoscopic low-profile trocar-cannula assembly (Curcillo low-profile ports [Karl Storz]) is inserted into the abdomen. The abdomen is insufflated using a pressure regulating mechanical insufflator. After brief abdominal exploration with a 30° telescope, 2 additional low-profile 5-mm trocar-cannula assemblies are inserted in a triangular fashion adjacent to the initial port. For the second and third low-profile trocar-cannula insertions, the abdomen is partially deinsufflated, which facilitates mobilization of the skin and soft tissue associated with the initial incision and enables a small soft tissue flap to be created for tunneling of the ports adjacent to the initial trocar. Using minimal blunt dissection, a tunnel is undermined 1-cm to 2-cm laterally and caudally on either side of the initial 5-mm trocar-cannula assembly using a Kelly hemostat. Through those tunneled paths, the 2 low-profile trocar-cannula assemblies are inserted through the abdominal wall into the peritoneal cavity using the sharp trocars under optical visualization. The 3 trocars are arranged in a deliberate triangular arrangement that causes

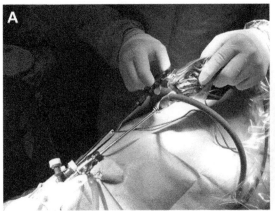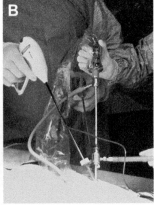

Fig. 5. Single-port access setup. (*A*) Once the initial 1.5-cm to 2-cm incision is made and the first 5-mm trocar is placed on midline, 2 more 5-mm trocars are placed 2 cm caudolateral to the first port. (*B*) The 3 ports are arranged in a triangular fashion.

the skin to stretch in a lateral direction. This arrangement enables each low-profile cannula to enter the abdomen through separate facial openings but through the same skin incision.

An advantage of this entry method is that it uses existing standard metal and reusable trocar-cannula assemblies, thus avoiding the cost associated with purchasing additional (often disposable) equipment.

INNOVATIVE ADAPTATIONS
Wound Retractor with Latex Glove and Finger Ports

A 2-cm to 3-cm minilaparotomy incision is created in advance for insertion of the port (**Fig. 6**). The inner ring of a 360° atraumatic wound retraction device (Alexis wound retractor [Applied Medical] and SurgiSleeve wound protector [Covidien]) is first inserted through the minilaparotomy incision. The outer ring is rolled until it reaches the level of the skin causing the retractor sheath to be pulled taught. The tips of the fingers of a sterile latex glove are cut to allow a 5-mm to 10-mm trocar-cannula assembly to be inserted. Suture is tied securely around the trocar-cannula assembly at the junction of the latex fingertip and the port. The wrist portion of the glove is then stretched over the external ring of the wound retractor. Insufflator tubing is attached to any of the finger port Luer-Lok fittings, and the abdomen is insufflated. All 5 fingers can be used as ports of entry if necessary.

Instrumentation and Optics

An array of articulating and prebent laparoscopic instruments has been developed and marketed specifically for the single-port platform in an effort to correct the difficulties inherent with the loss of triangulation (**Fig. 7**).[7,16,45,48] Bent or coaxial deviating instruments (coaxial instruments [Karl Storz]) are in a fixed position and are designed to be offset from the straight axis of a standard instrument.[48,49] This curved design

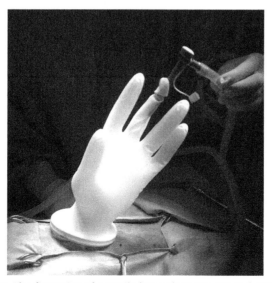

Fig. 6. Glove setup. The fingertips of a sterile latex glove are cut and attached to 5-mm to 10-mm trocar-cannula assemblies. The wrist portion of the glove is stretched over the external ring of a 360° wound retractor placed within a minilaparotomy incision.

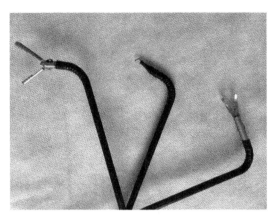

Fig. 7. Articulating graspers (Covidian) can be used through single-port devices and help facilitate adequate triangulation and minimize instrument collisions.

provides acceptable intracorporeal triangulation and good ergonomic position for the hands.[16] Double prebent instruments are intended to mimic triangulation through a curved design at both ends of the instrument shaft, which leads to antipodal directions of the tips and handles when the instruments are held parallel.[48] Articulating instruments (articulating grasper and scissors [Covidien]) have a design that mimics the movements of a surgeon's wrist and have a distal tip that can deflect relative to the instrument shaft.[7] Many of these instruments also offer axial 360° rotation for tip orientation similar to conventional rigid instruments.

All the articulating instruments can be introduced through single-port devices as well as conventional rigid trocar-cannula assemblies. In contrast, the double prebent instruments can only be used with soft, flexible, or specifically designed entry devices for bent instruments, because the bends in these instruments prevent their introduction into a rigid trocar-cannula assembly.

Due to the close proximity of the telescope and instruments during single-port laparoscopy, adjustments must be made to create enough working space for the surgeon, both intracorporeally and extracorporeally. Likely the easiest way to avoid instrument and optic interference is by using an angled telescope.[15,42,45] The most common telescope used for single-port laparoscopy in veterinary medicine is a telescope with a 30° lens. Recently, advanced laparoscopes specifically designed for single-port surgery have also emerged (EndoCAMeleon [Karl Storz], EndoEye [Olympus], and Ideal Eyes [Stryker, Kalamazoo, Michigan]).[50] Using a 30° or advanced deflecting telescope enables the telescope's camera head and tip to be directed away from the other instruments during single-port procedures, thus improving working space while simultaneously maintaining excellent visualization.[15,42,45,49]

SINGLE-PORT PROCEDURES
Ovariectomy

Indications
In most instances of ovarian disease, surgical removal of the diseased tissue by OVE is the recommended treatment.[50] Elective sterilization is the most common indication, however, for OVE in veterinary patients. Elective OVE significantly reduces the risk of mammary neoplasia in both dogs and cats, with the risk in dogs essentially nullified if surgery is performed before the first estrus.[51,52] Even older dogs, however, may

experience a reduced risk for mammary neoplasia when spayed later in life.[52] OVE also eliminates the risk of pyometra, which in many cases can be life threatening.[53–55] Some investigators suggest OVE may correct sexually dimorphic aggression in intact female dogs.[56]

Long-term studies have failed to show significant advantage of ovariohysterectomy compared with OVE alone.[54] Likewise, potential long-term complications associated with female sterilization, including urinary incontinence and obesity, are not significantly different between ovariohysterectomy and OVE.[50,54]

Contraindications
Laparoscopic OVE is unsuitable for patients with known uterine pathology (neoplasia or pyometra). Likewise, if uterine disease is identified at the time if initial laparoscopic exploration, conversion to an open approach is recommended. In the authors' experience, single-port OVE is more technically challenging in small patients (dogs or cats <10 kg) and, therefore, should be cautiously attempted by surgeons early in their learning curve.

Patient preparation and positioning
The patient is positioned in dorsal recumbency on a mechanical tilt table (C-Arms International, San Diego, California). The ventral aspect of the abdomen is clipped from the xiphoid to pubis for abdominal surgery, prepared for aseptic surgery, and draped for conventional open celiotomy to allow for additional trocar placement or conversion to open laparotomy if necessary.

Approach and port placement
A 2-cm to 3-cm skin incision is made at the level of the umbilicus. Dissection through the subcutaneous tissue and linea alba is performed using monopolar electrocautery or sharp dissection. A SILS Port is inserted into the incision, and the abdominal cavity is insufflated to 8 to 10 mm Hg with CO_2 using a pressure regulating mechanical insufflator (Endoflator [Karl Storz]). The multitrocar port is positioned with the three 5-mm cannulas at the 10-o'clock, 6-o'clock, and 2-o'clock positions to facilitate triangulation. A 5-mm 30° laparoscope (Hopkins II [Karl Storz]) is inserted into the 10 o'clock trocar and oriented caudally to view the abdomen and perform a limited abdominal explore.

Ovariectomy procedure
A technique for single-port laparoscopic OVE has been described by Manassero and colleagues[39] and Runge and colleagues[40] (Fig. 8). With the primary surgeon positioned on the right side of the patient, the mechanical tilt table is angled 30° to 45° to the right. A 30° telescope is inserted through the 10 o'clock cannula. A 5-mm articulating grasper (SILS Clinch XL [Covidien]) is inserted through the 2 o'clock cannula and positioned intra-abdominally to create a 90° positional bend at the distal third of the instrument with the tip deflecting toward the left ovary. The proper ligament is grasped and suspended with the articulating instrument. A 5-mm bipolar vessel sealing device (LigaSure V [Covidien]) is then inserted through the 6 o'clock cannula and directed toward the suspended left ovary. The ovarian artery and vein are grasped, sealed, and divided, followed by the remaining attachment of the mesovarium, including the suspensory ligament. The vessel sealing device is then directed and positioned just caudal to the proper ligament and the tissue sealed and divided at the level of the distal uterine horn. Once the ovarian tissue is freed and hemostasis confirmed, the vessel sealing device is removed. While still grasping the ovarian tissue, the articulating grasper is straightened and withdrawn into the multitrocar port. The camera is removed, insufflation stopped, and the 2 empty cannulas removed.

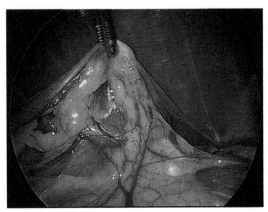

Fig. 8. During single-port laparoscopic OVE, an articulating grasper is used to suspend the ovary while a LigaSure device (Covidian) seals and transects the ovarian pedicle.

With the articulating grasper and left ovary within the remaining cannula, the external edge of the SILS Port is grasped digitally and removed from the abdominal incision. The dog is repositioned in dorsal recumbency and the multitrocar port is reinserted. The surgeon moves to the left side of the patient, and the procedure is repeated for removal of the right ovary. After completion of the OVE procedure, the incision is closed routinely in 3 layers.

Complications and management
Potential intraoperative complications associated with laparoscopic OVE include visceral trauma during port placement, hemorrhage from the ovarian pedicle, and loss of ovaries during their extraction.[6,39–41] Significant visceral trauma necessitates conversion to open laparotomy. Often, minor hemorrhage from the ovarian pedicle can be controlled by regrasping the pedicle and resealing the vessels using a vessel sealing device. If hemorrhage obscures the surgeon's field of view or cannot be controlled in a timely fashion, however, additional port placement or conversion to an open laparotomy is recommended. Ovaries lost during extraction are easily identified and regrasped using the telescope and articulating grasper, respectively, through the existing abdominal incision. Short-term incisional complications, including erythema, seroma, and infection, are uncommon and typically self-limiting, occurring at a frequency similar to that reported for other laparoscopic abdominal procedures.[39,40]

Postoperative care
Dogs are administered injectable nonsteroidal anti-inflammatory medication postoperatively. Dogs are administered injectable opioids postoperatively (methadone 0.1–0.2 mg/kg IV every 4–6 hours or buprenorphine 0.01 mg/kg IV every 6–8 hours) and hospitalized overnight as needed. Dogs can be discharged 8 to 12 hours after surgery on a 3-day to 5-day course of oral nonsteroidal anti-inflammatory medication and/or tramadol (2–4 mg/kg orally every 8–12 hours) based on clinician preference. All dogs are sent home with an Elizabethan collar, and 7 to 10 days of activity restriction is recommended.

Reporting, follow-up, and clinical implications
Excellent short-term and long-term outcomes have been documented for dogs undergoing laparoscopic OVE.[39–41] Perioperative complications are rare and similar to

those reported for other laparoscopic abdominal procedures.[6,39,40] In the most recent and largest study to date, no dogs that underwent laparoscopic sterilization were reported to have exhibited signs of heat or were diagnosed with a pyometra or ovarian remnant after surgery, thus validating the technique as an effective method for removal of all ovarian tissue.[57] The surgery time associated with single-port laparoscopic OVE has been reported significantly shorter than other laparoscopic techniques (ovariohysterectomy or multiport OVE).[57]

Ovariectomy in Combination with Gastropexy

Indications
Gastric dilatation and volvulus (GDV) is a life-threatening condition characterized by gastric dilatation, malpositioning of the stomach, and intra-abdominal venous obstruction resulting in reduced cardiac output and inadequate tissue perfusion.[58,59] Even with aggressive management and surgical intervention, the mortality rate for GDV is estimated to be between 10% and 30% and without a gastropexy the recurrence rate is greater than 50%.[60–64] Gastropexy, which creates a permanent adhesion of the stomach to the abdominal wall, is considered a standard of care adjunctive procedure that should be performed at the time of surgical GDV correction or as prophylaxis in predisposed breeds, dogs with a history of gastric dilatation, or dogs with a history of chronic volvulus.[59] Prophylactic laparoscopic-assisted gastropexy should be considered in a clinically stable dog at risk for GDV and can be easily performed concurrently with other elective laparoscopic procedures, including OVE, cryptorchidectomy, or organ biopsy.

Contraindications
Laparoscopic-assisted gastropexy should not be considered in dogs diagnosed with GDV or other significant intra-abdominal disease processes, because in these cases open laparotomy is the standard of care.

Patient preparation and positioning
The patient is positioned in dorsal recumbency on a mechanical tilt table (C-Arms International), and the abdomen is clipped and prepped from xiphoid to pubis. Care should be taken to ensure the clip job extends a sufficient amount along the right lateral body wall.

Approach and port placement
The single-port access laparoscopic gastropexy was originally described by Runge and Mayhew[41] (**Fig. 9**). Briefly, a 2-cm to 3-cm skin incision is made starting just lateral to the rectus abdominus muscle and 2-cm to 5-cm caudal to the right 13th rib. Dissection through the oblique and transverse abdominal musculature is continued using a combination of monopolar electrocautery and sharp dissection. Stay sutures are placed in the cauterized/cut edges of the transversus abdominus muscle, and a SILS with three 5-mm cannulas is inserted. Insufflator tubing is attached to the SILS insufflation port and the abdomen is insufflated to 8 to 10 mm Hg with CO_2. A 5-mm 30° laparoscope (Hopkins II) is inserted into a cannula and oriented caudally for a limited abdominal explore.

Spay and gastropexy procedure
Laparoscopic OVE is performed as described previously. Once ovaries have been removed by exteriorization of the SILS device, the port is reinserted through the same incision. Two 5-mm cannulas and one 12-mm cannula are inserted and the abdomen is reinsufflated. The table may be tilted in a slight reverse Trendelenburg

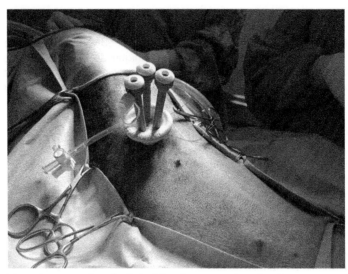

Fig. 9. Incision placement for single-incision laparoscopic-assisted gastropexy. A 2-cm to 3-cm minilaparotomy is positioned just lateral to the rectus abdominus muscle and 2-cm to 5-cm incision caudal to the right 13th rib.

position to facilitate exposure of the greater curvature of the stomach. A 30° telescope is inserted into one of the 5-mm cannulas, and standard rigid 10-mm DuVal forceps are inserted through the cannula and directed toward the antrum of the stomach. A relatively avascular region near the antrum is grasped atraumatically midway between the greater and lesser curvatures for use as the gastropexy site. Holding firmly with the forceps, the stomach is carefully exteriorized by first removing the telescope followed by the two 5-mm cannulas. As insufflation is lost, the SILS Port is removed while still grasping the stomach. The stomach is exteriorized through the abdominal incision, and stay sutures are placed to maintain orientation of the gastric axis. An incisional gastropexy is performed as described by Rawlings and colleagues[35] for conventional laparoscopic-assisted incisional gastropexy. The body wall is closed in individual muscle layers, followed by the subcutaneous tissue and skin.

Complications and management
Potential complications of laparoscopic OVE in combination with laparoscopic-assisted gastropexy are similar for those listed previously for laparoscopic OVE. Additionally, inaccurate port placement (too lateral) may result in poor visualization of the left ovary and prolonged procedure time.[41] Seroma formation is not uncommon with the gastropexy procedure but is typically self-limiting. It is the authors' opinion that careful closure of the body wall in individual muscle layers helps reduce seroma incidence.

Postoperative care
Dogs are administered injectable opioids postoperatively (methadone 0.1–0.2 mg/kg IV every 4–6 hours or buprenorphine 0.01 mg/kg IV every 6–8 hours) and hospitalized overnight. Dogs are discharged the day after surgery on a 5-day course of nonsteroidal anti-inflammatory medication and/or tramadol (2–4 mg/kg orally every 8–12 hours) based on clinician preference. An Elizabethan collar and activity restriction are recommended for 14 days postoperatively. Lifelong medical management strategies to prevent gastric dilatation should be discussed with clients.

Reporting, follow-up, and clinical implications

Laparoscopic-assisted gastropexy has proved an effective minimally invasive method of preventing GDV in predisposed breeds.[65–67] Rawlings[65] reported on the long-term success of the technique by following surgically treated dogs 1 year postoperatively. In this study, no dogs were diagnosed with GDV during the study period, and ultrasonographic evaluation performed 1 year after surgery confirmed persistent attachment between the stomach and abdominal wall. Long-term complications associated with gastropexy, including persistent or intermittent signs of gastric upset or gastric outflow obstruction have been infrequently reported, and it is the authors' opinion that the risk of such signs can be minimized by ensuring appropriate gastropexy positioning.

Cryptorchidectomy

Indications

Cryptorchidectomy is recommended for removal of undescended testes, because they are 13.6 times as likely to develop neoplasia and are also at an increased risk of torsion when compared to descended testes.[68,69] Traditionally, open abdominal exploration was performed for identification and removal of nonpalpable testes is veterinary patients.[70,71] This was followed by a description of multiport laparoscopic cryptorchidectomy, which was less invasive than open laparotomy but required multiple incisions for port placement as well as incision elongation for tissue removal.[38,72–75] Even more recently, Runge and colleagues[45] have described a technique for single-port laparoscopic cryptorchidectomy.

Contraindications

In patients presenting with an acute abdomen due to torsion of the cryptorchid testicle or in patients with concurrent intra-abdominal disease necessitating thorough exploration, open laparotomy should be considered over a minimally invasive approach. Likewise, the presence of significant adhesions between the retained testicle(s) and other abdominal contents identified at the time of initial laparoscopic exploration may necessitate conversion to open laparotomy.

Patient preparation and positioning

The patient is positioned in dorsal recumbency and the ventral abdomen from xiphoid to pubis is clipped and aseptically prepped. Prior to the procedure, the urinary bladder is manually expressed to ensure ample working space in the caudal aspect of the abdomen. Ideally, a mechanical tilt table is used so the patient can be positioned laterally or in a Trendelenburg position to facilitate the procedure.

Approach and port placement

A 1.5-cm to 3-cm ventral midline incision is made at the level of the umbilicus through the skin, subcutaneous tissue, and body wall using a combination of sharp dissection and electrocautery. A SILS Port, EndoCone, or TriPort can be introduced into the abdominal incision to complete the single-port procedure. The abdomen is insufflated to 8 to 10 mm Hg with CO_2.

Cryptorchidectomy procedure

A 30° telescope (Hopkins II) is positioned through the single-port device to visualize the caudal abdomen. A 5-mm articulating grasper (SILS Clinch XL) is used to manipulate tissue and locate the testis. The testis is then grasped and elevated with the articulating instrument, enabling visualization of the vascular pedicle, spermatic cord, and gubernaculum. A laparoscopic bipolar vessel sealing device (LigaSure V) is inserted through the port into the abdomen and used to seal and transect the vascular pedicle, spermatic cord, and gubernaculum, in that order. The resected testis is maintained within the grasp of the forceps and brought to the base of the port under direct visualization. The telescope is removed, followed by the 2 empty cannulas. As pneumoperitoneum is lost, the port is removed along with the forceps containing the resected testis. The incision is then closed routinely.

Complications and management
Potential complications associated with laparoscopic cryptorchidectomy are similar to those reported for laparoscopic OVE and managed in similar fashion. Given the incidence of neoplasia diagnosed in cryptorchid testicles, histopathologic evaluation is recommended.

Postoperative care
Patients are administered injectable nonsteroidal anti-inflammatory medication postoperatively. Dogs can be administered injectable opioids postoperatively (methadone 0.1–0.2 mg/kg IV every 4–6 hours or buprenorphine 0.01 mg/kg IV every 6–8 hours) and hospitalized overnight if needed. A majority of patients can be discharged the evening of the procedure (6–12 hours postoperatively) on a 3-day to 5-day course of oral nonsteroidal anti-inflammatory medication and/or tramadol (2–4 mg/kg orally every 8–12 hours) based on clinician preference. An Elizabethan collar and 7 to 10 days of activity restriction are recommended.

Reporting, follow-up, and clinical implications
In the 1 study to date describing the perioperative outcome of single-port laparoscopic cryptorchidectomy in dogs and cats, successful removal of the undescended testis was performed in all cases, and no intraoperative complications were encountered.[45] Proposed benefits of the single-port cryptorchidectomy compared with open laparotomy or multiport laparoscopic cryptorchidectomy include the necessity for only a single abdominal incision, the ability to treat patients with bilateral disease without the need for additional incisions, and ease of specimen retrieval at any point during the procedure with quick re-establishment of pneumoperitoneum.[45,75] Additionally, the procedure can be performed safely in both canine and feline patients of varying body weight.[45]

Hepatic biopsy

Indications
Liver biopsy is indicated for dogs and cats with diffuse or multifocal hepatic disease to provide a histologic diagnosis which, in turn, guides prognosis and recommended therapy (**Fig. 10**).[76] Laparoscopic liver biopsy provides the benefits of a minimally invasive surgery while allowing the surgeon to obtain multiple, representative samples under direct visualization, thus maximizing the diagnostic potential of the procedure.[77]

Contraindications
Few true contraindications exist for laparoscopic liver biopsy, as long as the patient is stable enough to undergo general anesthesia. A recent study by McDevitt and colleagues[44] has documented the procedure to be safe and effective even in cases of advanced liver disease and coagulopathy. Ascites has been considered a relative contraindication to laparoscopy in both veterinary and human patients, because abdominal fluid may inhibit adequate visualization.[78] In the authors' opinion, however, laparoscopic liver biopsy can still be performed in the presence of ascites, because abdominal fluid can be removed via suction if necessary to allow sufficient visualization during the procedure.

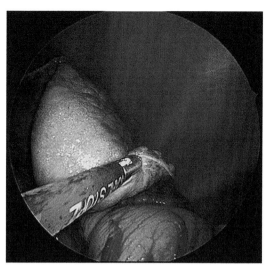

Fig. 10. Single-port laparoscopic liver biopsy; 5-mm biopsy cup forceps are introduced through a 5-mm SILS cannula (SILS Port) and used to grasp a representative sample of hepatic parenchyma. The tissue is twisted 360° for 4 to 6 revolutions prior to removal to stimulate vascular spasm and minimize bleeding.

Patient preparation and positioning

The patient is positioned in dorsal recumbency, ideally on a mechanical tilt table. The abdomen is clipped and prepped from 2 cm cranial to the xiphoid caudally to the pubis.

Approach and port placement

A 2-cm incision is made through the skin, subcutaneous tissue, and body wall using a combination of sharp dissection and monopolar electrocautery. A SILS Port is introduced through the abdominal incision with three 5-mm cannulas. The abdomen is insufflated to an intra-abdominal pressure of 8 to 10 mm Hg using a pressure regulating mechanical insufflator.

Laparoscopic liver biopsy technique

The technique for single-port laparoscopic liver biopsy has been recently described by McDevitt and collegues.[44] In summary, a 5-mm 30° telescope (Hopkins II) is inserted through 1 of the SILS cannulas, and a limited abdominal explore is performed noting presence of ascites, gross hepatic appearance, and/or other abdominal pathology. A 5-mm blunt laparoscopic probe is then introduced through one of the cannulas and, under direct visualization, used to manipulate each of the liver lobes such that both the diaphragmatic and peritoneal surfaces are adequately evaluated for disease. If necessary, the patient can be tilted to facilitate visualization of all liver lobes. The blunt probe is then removed from the abdomen and replaced with 5-mm biopsy cup forceps, which are used to obtain 3 to 5 tissue biopsies from representative lesions along the periphery of the liver lobes. This is achieved by grasping the tissue with the biopsy forceps and twisting in a clockwise fashion for 4 to 6 full revolutions on the instrument shaft axis. Traction is applied until the specimen is free from the surrounding hepatic parenchyma. The specimen is removed from the abdomen, and the procedure is repeated until all samples are obtained. The biopsy sites are examined for any evidence of continued or excessive hemorrhage. The SILS Port is then removed, and the incision is closed routinely.

Complications and management

Reported complications of the laparoscopic liver biopsy are similar to other laparoscopic abdominal procedures, namely visceral trauma during port placement.[77,79] Prolonged or excessive hemorrhage from the biopsy sites is rare in the authors' experience, even in patients with known bleeding disorders, as long as appropriate perioperative medical therapies are prescribed.[44] If minor, persistent bleeding is noted from the biopsy sites, hemostatic agents can be gently placed over the areas of concern. If excessive hemorrhage is noted, conversion to open laparotomy is recommended.

Postoperative care

Patients are administered injectable analgesia (methadone 0.1–0.2 mg/kg IV every 4–6 hours or buprenorphine 0.01 mg/kg IV every 6–8 hours) postoperatively. Patients are hospitalized overnight or longer, depending on the severity of underlying hepatic disease, and monitored for clinical signs or clinicopathologic derangements suggestive of intra-abdominal bleeding. Patients are discharged on a 3 to 5 day course of tramadol (2–4 mg/kg IV every 8–12 hours), with an Elizabethan collar and instructions for 7 to 10 days of activity restriction.

Reporting, follow-up, and clinical implications

Laparoscopic liver biopsy has been proved a safe and effective minimally invasive technique for obtaining hepatic tissue samples of diagnostic quality.[44,77,79] In the most recent study to date evaluating the safety and efficacy of laparoscopic hepatic biopsy in companion animals, a complication rate of 1.9% was described; this study included patients of varying sizes as well as patients with clinical signs of advanced liver disease, including coagulopathy, thrombocytopenia, and ascites.[44] There is currently a paucity of data objectively comparing the single-port laparoscopic biopsy with the more conventional multiport technique, which is certainly a topic for future research.

Laparoscopic-assisted Intestinal Surgery

Indications

Single-incision laparoscopic-assisted intestinal surgery (SILAIS)—biopsy, enterotomy, resection, and anastomosis—is indicated for the diagnosis and treatment of stabile dogs and cats with small intestinal disease including but not limited to inflammatory bowel disease, infiltrative/neoplastic disease, or foreign body obstruction.[78,80,81]

Contraindications

This procedure should be not be considered for animals with evidence of peritonitis or visceral rupture.[42]

Patient preparation and positioning

The patient is positioned in dorsal recumbency, ideally on a mechanical tilt table. The ventral aspect of the abdomen is clipped from the xiphoid to pubis for abdominal surgery, prepared for aseptic surgery, and draped for conventional open laparotomy to allow for additional trocar placement or conversion to open surgery if necessary.

Approach and port placement

A 2-cm to 3-cm ventral midline skin incision is made just caudal to the umbilicus and continued through the linea alba. A SILS Port or EndoCone is inserted into the incision, and the peritoneal cavity is insufflated to 8 to 10 mm Hg with CO_2 gas.

Intestinal surgery

SILAIS has been described in detail by Case and Ellison[42] (**Fig. 11**). To summarize, a 5-mm 30° telescope is used for abdominal exploration. During exploration, the patient

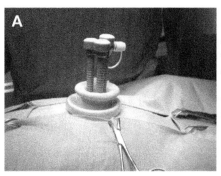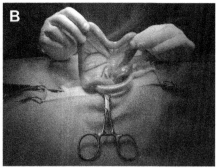

Fig. 11. Use of a wound retractor device (Alexis wound retractor and SurgiSleeve wound protector) in combination with a SILS Port for minimally invasive abdominal exploration with intestinal surgery. (*A*) After laparoscopic explore, the SILS Port can be removed for extracorporeal running of the small intestines. (*B*) The wound retractor device facilitates exteriorization of the bowel and provides a clean working surface.

may be tilted to facilitate examination of the abdominal gutters, and a blunt probe can be used to palpate and manipulate and gastrointestinal tract. A loop of jejunum is grasped using laparoscopic Babcock forceps and brought to the SILS Port, which is then gently removed. For the EndoCone, the bulkhead cap is removed and a section of jejunum digitally grasped. Moist laparotomy sponges are placed along the incision edge, and the small bowel is run extracorporeally in an orad direction to the level of the caudal duodenal flexure and aborally to the ileocolic junction, to ensure the site(s) of pathology are identified. Extracorporeal biopsy, enterotomy, or resection/anastomosis is performed using standard techniques. After the bowel is replaced into the abdomen, omentalization can be performed by grasping the greater omentum with laparoscopic Babcock forceps and wrapping it around the surgical site. The incision is then closed routinely.

Complications and management
Potential complications associated with laparoscopic-assisted intestinal surgery are similar for other laparoscopic abdominal procedures and intestinal surgery by laparotomy.[42,78,80,81] Inability to exteriorize the affected bowel or the presence of intra-abdominal adhesions may necessitate conversion to laparotomy or enlargement of the incision.[42] In the authors' experience, placement of a wound retractor device (Alexis wound retractor and SurgiSleeve wound protector) through the abdominal incision prior to placement of the SILS Port facilitates extracorporeal manipulation of the bowel.[43]

Postoperative care Postoperative management is dependent on a patient's clinical signs and severity of gastrointestinal disease. IV fluid therapy should is administered to maintain adequate hydration if clinically indicated, and injectable analgesia is continued for 24 to 48 hours postoperatively (methadone 0.1–0.2 mg/kg IV every 4–6 hours or buprenorphine 0.01 mg/kg IV every 6–8 hours). Gastrointestinal protectants and/or antiemetics may be administered based on clinician preference. Patients are offered water and small amounts of a bland diet 8 to 12 hours after surgery. Once patients are eating and drinking voluntarily without signs of gastrointestinal upset, they can be transitioned to oral pain medication (tramadol 2–4 mg/kg orally every 8–12 hours) and discharged from the hospital. An Elizabethan collar and 10 to 14 days of activity restriction are recommended.

Reporting, follow-up, and clinical implications

Case and Ellison[42] reported a good short-term postoperative outcome in all patients who underwent SILAIS for small intestinal disease, with no major perioperative complications encountered. No studies to date, however, have objectively compared SILAIS to other laparoscopic-assisted intestinal surgical techniques or intestinal surgery by laparotomy. Given that the accuracy of SILAIS for identification of small bowel pathology is currently unknown and abdominal exploration with SILAIS is limited, the authors stress the importance of thorough preoperative diagnostic imaging to confirm the presence and location of small intestinal disease.

SUMMARY

The single-port platform is a recent innovation in minimally invasive techniques and represents the next step toward scarless surgery. Early reports in the veterinary literature have show this access technique to be a safe, feasible, and potentially more attractive approach to a variety of common abdominal procedures.[39–45] As with all emerging surgical techniques, attention should be focused on procedural feasibility, safety, and efficacy. Additionally, the clinical advantage of the technique over other established methods should be clearly elucidated. Further studies are still needed to determine if the single-port platform can be considered a comparable alternative to multiport laparoscopy.

REFERENCES

1. Davidson EB, Moll HD, Payton ME. Comparison of laparoscopic ovariohysterectomy and ovariohysterectomy in dogs. Vet Surg 2004;33:62–9.
2. Devitt CM, Cox RE, Hailey JJ. Duration, complications, stress, and pain of open ovariohysterectomy versus a simple method of laparoscopic-assisted ovariohysterectomy in dogs. J Am Vet Med Assoc 2005;227:921–7.
3. Walsh PJ, Remendios AM, Ferguson JF, et al. Thoracoscopic versus open partial pericardectomy in dogs: comparison of postoperative pain and morbidity. Vet Surg 1999;28:472–9.
4. Culp WT, Mayhew PD, Brown DC. The effect of laparoscopic versus open ovariectomy on postsurgical activity in small dogs. Vet Surg 2009;38:811–7.
5. Karayiannakis AJ, Makri GG, Mantzioka A, et al. Postoperative pulmonary function after laparoscopic and open cholecystectomy. Br J Anaesth 1996;77:448–52.
6. Lansdowne JL, Mehler SJ, Boure LP. Minimally invasive abdominal and thoracic surgery: principles and instrumentation. Compend Contin Educ Vet 2012;34:E1–9.
7. Kommu SS, Rane A. Devices for laparoendoscopic single-site surgery in urology. Expert Rev Med Devices 2009;6:95–103.
8. Islam A, Castellvi AO, Tesfay ST, et al. Early surgeon impressions and technical difficulty associated with laparoendoscopic single-site surgery: a society of American gastrointestinal and endoscopic surgeons learning center study. Surg Endosc 2011;8:2597–603.
9. Galvao Neto M, Ramos A, Campos J. Single port laparoscopic access surgery. Gastrointest Endosc 2009;11:84–93.
10. Qiu J, Yuan H, Chen S, et al. Single-port versus conventional multiport laparoscopic cholecystectomy: a meta-analysis of randomized controlled trials and nonrandomized studies. J Laparoendosc Adv Surg Tech A 2013;23:815–31.
11. Podolsky ER, Curcillo PG. Single Port Access (SPA) Surgery—a 24-Month Experience. J Gastrointest Surg 2010;14:759–67.

12. Fader AN, Levinson KL, Gunderson CC, et al. Laparoendoscopic single-site surgery in gynaecology. A new frontier in minimally invasive surgery. J Minim Access Surg 2011;7:71–7.
13. Mencaglia L, Mereu L, Carri G, et al. Single-port entry—are there any advantages? Best Pract Res Clin Obstet Gynaecol 2013;3:441–55.
14. Antoniou SA, Koch OO, Antoniou G. Meta-analysis of randomized trials on single-incision laparoscopic versus conventional laparoscopic appendectomy. Am J Surg 2014;207:613–22.
15. Runge JJ. The cutting edge: introducing reduced port laparoscopic surgery. Today's Veterinary Practice 2012;14–20.
16. Rieder E, Martinec DV, Cassera MA, et al. A triangulating operating platform enhances bimanual performance and reduces surgical workload in single-incision laparoscopy. J Am Coll Surg 2011;212:378–84.
17. Ahmed MU, Aftab A, Seriwala HM, et al. Can single incision laparoscopic cholecystectomy replace the traditional four port laparoscopic approach: a review. Glob J Health Sci 2014;15:119–25.
18. Chang SK, Lee KY. Therapeutic advances: single incision laparoscopic hepatopancreatobiliary surgery. World J Gastroenterol 2014;20:14329–37.
19. Sinha R, Yadav AS. Transumbilical single incision laparoscopic cholecystectomy with conventional instruments: a continuing study. J Minim Access Surg 2014;10:175–9.
20. Hirano D, Hasegawa R, Igarashi T, et al. Laparoscopic adrenalectomy for adrenal tumors: a 21-year single-institution experience. Asian J Surg 2014;38:79–84.
21. Vidal O, Astudillo E, Valentini M, et al. Single-port laparoscopic left adrenalectomy (SILS): 3 year's experience of a single institution. Surg Laparosc Endosc Percutan Tech 2014;24:440–3.
22. Gurluler E, Berber I, Cakir U, et al. Laparoendoscopic single-site donor nephrectomy: a single-center initial experience. Ann Transplant 2014;19:551–5.
23. Barth RN, Phelan MW, Goldschen L, et al. Single-port donor nephrectomy provides improved patient satisfaction and equivalent outcomes. Ann Surg 2013;257:527–33.
24. Liang HH, Hung CS, Wang W, et al. Single-incision versus conventional laparoscopic appendectomy in 688 patients: a retrospective comparative analysis. Can J Surg 2014;57:E89–97.
25. Al Sabah S, Liberman AS, Wongyingsinn M, et al. Single-port laparoscopic colorectal surgery: early clinical experience. J Laparoendosc Adv Surg Tech A 2012;22:853–7.
26. Yoon BS, Seong SJ, Kim IH, et al. Operative outcomes of single-port-access laparoscopy-assisted vaginal hysterectomy compared with single-port-access total laparoscopic hysterectomy. Taiwan J Obstet Gynecol 2014;53:486–9.
27. Kim SM, Park EK, Jeung IC, et al. Abdominal, multi-port and single-port total laparoscopic hysterectomy: eleven-year trends comparison of surgical outcomes complications of 936 cases. Arch Gynecol Obstet 2015;291(6):1313–9.
28. Song T, Lee SH. Barbed suture vs traditional suture in single-port total laparoscopic hysterectomy. J Minim Invasive Gynecol 2014;21:825–9.
29. Yang YS, Kim SY, Hur MH, et al. Natural orifice transluminal endoscopic surgery-assisted versus single-port laparoscopic-assisted vaginal hysterectomy: a case-matched study. J Minim Invasive Gynecol 2014;21:624–31.
30. Gao X, Pang J, Situ J, et al. Single-port transvesical laparoscopic radical prostatectomy for organ-confined prostate cancer: technique and outcomes. BJU Int 2013;112:944–52.

31. Kaouk JH, Goel RK, Haber GP, et al. Single-port laparoscopic radical prostatectomy. Urology 2008;72:1190–3.
32. Tsujihata M, Miyake O, Yoshimura K, et al. Laparoscopic diagnosis and treatment of nonpalpable testis. Int J Urol 2001;8:692–6.
33. Bansal D, Cost NG, Bean CM, et al. Pediatric urological laparoendoscopic single site surgery: Single surgeon experience. J Pediatr Urol 2014;10:1170–5.
34. Pucher PH, Sodergren MH, Singh P, et al. Have we learned from lessons of the past? A systematic review of training for single incision laparoscopic surgery. Surg Endosc 2012;27:1478–84.
35. Rawlings C, Foutz TL, Mahaffey MB, et al. A rapid and strong laparoscopic-assisted gastropexy in dogs. Am J Vet Res 2011;62:871–5.
36. Rawlings CA, Howerth EW, Mahaffery MB, et al. Laparoscopic-assisted cystopexy in dogs. Am J Vet Res 2002;63:1226–31.
37. Rawlings CA, Mahaffey MB, Barsanti JA, et al. Use of laparoscopic-assisted cystoscopy for removal of urinary calculi in dogs. J Am Vet Med Assoc 2003;222:759–61.
38. Miller NA, Van Lue SJ, Rawlings CA. Use of laparoscopic-assisted cryptorchidectomy in dogs and cats. J Am Vet Med Assoc 2004;224:875–8.
39. Manassero M, Leperlier D, Vallefuoco R, et al. Laparoscopic ovariectomy in dogs using a single-port multiple-access device. Vet Rec 2012;171:69.
40. Runge JJ, Curcillo PG II, King SA, et al. Initial application of reduced port surgery using the single port access technique for laparoscopic canine ovariectomy. Vet Surg 2012;41:803–6.
41. Runge JJ, Mayhew PD. Evaluation of single port access gastropexy and ovariectomy using articulating instruments and angled telescopes in dogs. Vet Surg 2013;42:807–13.
42. Case JB, Ellison G. Single incision laparoscopic-assisted intestinal surgery (SILAIS) in 7 dogs and 1 cat. Vet Surg 2013;42:629–34.
43. Baron JK, Giuffrida MA, Mayhew P, et al. Evaluation of minimally invasive abdominal exploration and intestinal biopsies (MIAEB) using a novel wound retraction device in cats: 31 cases (2005-2013). Abstract Presented at the ACVS Surgery Summit. San Diego, October 15–18, 2014.
44. McDevitt H, Brown D, Giuffrida M, et al. Complications and conversion rates associated with laparoscopic liver biopsies in dogs: 106 cases (2005-2013). Abstract Presented at the ACVS Surgery Summit. San Diego, October 15–18, 2014.
45. Runge JJ, Mayhew PD, Case JB, et al. Single-port laparoscopic cryptorchidectomy in dogs and cats: 25 cases (2009-2014). J Am Vet Med Assoc 2014;245(11):1258–65.
46. Runge JJ, Boston RC, Ross SB, et al. Evaluation of the learning curve for a board-certified veterinary surgeon performing laparoendoscopic single-site ovariectomy in dogs. In: Proceedings of the 9th Annual Meeting of the Veterinary Endoscopy Society. Park City, March 22–24, 2012.
47. Coisman JG, Case JB, Clark ND, et al. Efficacy of decontamination and sterilization of a single-use single-incision laparoscopic surgery port. Am J Vet Res 2013;74:934–8.
48. Miernik A, Schoenthaler M, Lilienthal K, et al. Pre-bent instruments used in single-port laparoscopic surgery versus conventional laparoscopic surgery: comparative study of performance in a dry lab. Surg Endosc 2012;26:1924–30.
49. Goldsmith ZG, Astroza GM, Wang AJ, et al. Optical performance comparison of deflectable laparoscopies for laparoendoscopic single-site surgery. J Endourol 2012;26:1340–5.

50. Fransson BA. Ovaries and uterus. In: Tobias K, Johnston S, editors. Veterinary surgery: small animal. St. Louis (MO): Elsevier; 2011. p. 1871–902.
51. Overly B, Shofer FS, Goldschmidt MH, et al. Association between ovariohysterectomy and feline mammary carcinoma. J Vet Intern Med 2005;19:560–3.
52. Schneider R, Dorn CR, Taylor DO. Factors influencing canine mammary cancer development and postsurgical survival. J Natl Cancer Inst 1969;43:1249–61.
53. Egenvall A, Hagman R, Bonnett BN, et al. Breed risk of pyometra in insured dogs in Sweden. J Vet Intern Med 2001;15:530–8.
54. Van Goethem B, Schaefers-Okkens A, Kirpensteijn J. Making a rational choice between ovariectomy and ovariohysterectomy in the dog: a discussion of the benefits of either technique. Vet Surg 2006;35:136–43.
55. Hagman R, Reezigt BJ, Bergstrom Ledin H, et al. Blood lactate levels in 31 female dogs with pyometra. Acta Vet Scand 2009;51:2.
56. Kustritz MV. Determining the optimal age for gonadectomy of dogs and cats. J Am Vet Med Assoc 2007;231:1665–75.
57. Corriveau KM, Giuffrida M, Runge J. Comparison of ovariectomy and ovariohysterectomy for canine laparoscopic sterilization. Abstract Presented at the ACVS Surgery Summit. San Diego, October 15–18, 2014.
58. Aronson LR, Brockman DJ, Brown DC. Gastrointestinal emergencies. Vet Clin North Am Small Anim Pract 2000;30:555–79.
59. Burrows CG, Ignaszewski A. Canine gastric dilation-volvulus. J Small Anim Pract 1990;31:495–501.
60. Brockman JD, Washabau RJ, Drobatz KJ. Canine gastric dilation-volvulus syndrome in a veterinary critical care unit: 295 cases (1986-1992). J Am Vet Med Assoc 1995;207:460–4.
61. Glickman LT, Glickman NW, Perez CM, et al. Analysis of risk factors for gastric dilation and dilation-volvulus in dogs. J Am Vet Med Assoc 1994;204:1965–71.
62. Glickman LT, Lantz GC, Schellenberg DB, et al. A prospective study of survival and recurrence following the acute gastric dilation-volvulus syndrome in 136 dogs. J Am Anim Hosp Assoc 1998;34:253–9.
63. Beck JJ, Staatz AJ, Pelsue DH, et al. Risk factors associated with short-term outcome and development of perioperative complications in dogs undergoing surgery because of gastric-dilation-volvulus: 166 cases (1992-2003). J Am Vet Med Assoc 2006;229:1934–9.
64. Mackenzie G, Barnhart M, Kennedy S, et al. A retrospective study of factors influencing survival following surgery for gastric dilatation-volvulus syndrome in 306 dogs. J Am Anim Hosp Assoc 2010;46:97–102.
65. Rawlings CA. Laparoscopic-assisted gastropexy. J Am Anim Hosp Assoc 2002; 38:15–9.
66. Runge J, Mayhew P, Rawlings CA. Laparoscopic-assisted and laparoscopic prophylactic gastropexy: indications and techniques. Compend Contin Educ Vet 2009;31:58–65.
67. Rawlings CA, Mahaffey MB, Bement S, et al. Prospective evaluation of laparoscopic-assisted gastropexy in dogs susceptible to gastric dilatation. J Am Vet Med Assoc 2002;221:1576–81.
68. Hayes HM, Pendergrass TW. Canine testicular tumors: epidemiologic features of 410 dogs. Int J Cancer 1976;18:482–7.
69. Pendergrass TW, Hayes HM. Cryptorchism and related defects in dogs: epidemiologic comparisons with man. Teratology 1975;12:51–5.
70. Booth HW. Testis and epididymis. In: Slatter D, editor. Textbook of small animal surgery. 3rd edition. Philadelphia: Saunders; 2002. p. 1521–7.

71. Gradili C, McCarthy R. Cryptorchidism. In: Monnet E, editor. Textbook of small animal soft tissue surgery. Ames (IA): John Wiley & Sons; 2012. p. 681–5.

72. Dunn ML, Foster WJ, Goddard KM. Cryptorchidism in dogs: a clinical survey. J Am Anim Hosp Assoc 1968;4:180–2.

73. Gimbo A, Catone G, Cristarella S, et al. A new, less invasive, laparoscopic-laparotomic technique for the cryptorchidectomy in the dog. Arch Ital Urol Androl 1993;65:277–81.

74. Spinella G, Romangnoli N, Valentini S, et al. Application of the 'extraction bag' in laparoscopic treatment of unilateral and bilateral abdominal cryptorchidism in dogs. Vet Res Commun 2003;27:445–7.

75. Mayhew P. Laparoscopic and laparoscopic-assisted cryptorchidectomy in dogs and cats. Compend Contin Educ Vet 2009;31:274–81.

76. Rothuizen J, Twedt D. Liver biopsy techniques. Vet Clin North Am Small Anim Pract 2009;37:469–80.

77. Petre S, Kovak-McClaran J, Bergman P, et al. Safety and efficacy of laparoscopic hepatic biopsy in dogs: 80 cases (22004-2009). J Am Vet Med Assoc 2012;240:181–5.

78. Freeman LJ. Gastrointestinal laparoscopy in small animals. Vet Clin North Am Small Anim Pract 2009;39:903–24.

79. Monet E, Twedt D. Laparoscopy. Vet Clin North Am Small Anim Pract 2003;33:1147–63.

80. Rawlings CA, Howerth EW, Bement S, et al. Laparoscopic-assisted enterostomy tube placement and full-thickness biopsy of the jejunum with serosal patching in dogs. Am J Vet Res 2002;63:1313–9.

81. Gower SB, Mayhew PD. A wound retraction device for laparoscopic-assisted intestinal surgery in dogs and cats. Vet Surg 2011;40:485–8.

Advances in Flexible Endoscopy

Anant Radhakrishnan, DVM

KEYWORDS

- Flexible endoscopy • Minimally invasive procedures • Gastroduodenoscopy
- Minimally invasive surgery

KEY POINTS

- Although some therapeutic uses exist, flexible endoscopy is primarily used as a diagnostic tool.
- Several novel flexible endoscopic procedures have been studied recently and show promise in veterinary medicine.
- These procedures provide the clinician with increased diagnostic capability.
- As the demand for minimally invasive procedures continues to increase, flexible endoscopy is being more readily investigated for therapeutic uses.
- The utility of flexible endoscopy in small animal practice should increase in the future with development of the advanced procedures summarized herein.

INTRODUCTION

The demand for minimally invasive therapeutic measures continues to increase in human and veterinary medicine. Pet owners are increasingly aware of technology and diagnostic options and often desire the same care for their pet that they may receive if hospitalized. Certain diseases, such as neoplasia, hepatobiliary disease, pancreatic disease, and gastric dilatation–volvulus, can have significant morbidity associated with them such that aggressive, invasive measures may be deemed unacceptable. Even less severe chronic illnesses such as inflammatory bowel disease can be associated with frustration for the pet owner such that more immediate and detailed information regarding their pet's disease may prove to be beneficial. Minimally invasive procedures that can increase diagnostic and therapeutic capability with reduced patient morbidity will be in demand and are therefore an area of active investigation.

The author has nothing to disclose.
Department of Internal Medicine, Bluegrass Veterinary Specialists + Animal Emergency, 1591 Winchester Road, Suite 106, Lexington, KY 40505, USA
E-mail address: anturad@yahoo.com

INDICATIONS

Flexible endoscopy is a versatile tool that provides visualization of the gastrointestinal lumen. During the procedure, samples are obtained to provide greater diagnostic information. Endoscopy is commonly used for the patient with gastrointestinal signs (**Box 1**), because other diagnostic tests such as complete blood count, serum chemistry, radiography, and ultrasonography may not provide definitive information to diagnose the underlying condition. The typical objectives of the endoscopist include visual evaluation of the mucosal surface of the stomach, small intestine, and large intestine for lesions such as ulcers or masses, and obtaining mucosal samples for histopathology, cytology, or culture. Flexible endoscopy can be of therapeutic value in several situations, such as gastric or esophageal foreign bodies, esophageal strictures, and feeding tube placement.

EQUIPMENT
Endoscope Components

Equipment and routine flexible endoscopic procedures have been described previously and are reviewed.[1] The typical flexible endoscope can be divided into 3 components: the handpiece, the insertion tube, and the umbilical cord (**Fig. 1**). The handpiece (**Fig. 2**) contains the main control mechanisms for the endoscope. For a fiberoptic scope, the eyepiece for visualization is on the end of the handpiece. A coupler can be attached to the eyepiece to accept a camera head for viewing on a monitor. For a flexible video endoscope, the handpiece does not contain an eyepiece. Control options include deflection of the insertion tube tip, insufflation, water infusion, and suction.

The insertion tube is the flexible portion of the endoscope that is inserted into the gastrointestinal tract for examination (**Fig. 3**). It contains channels for insufflation, water

---

Box 1
Common indications for gastrointestinal endoscopy

Abdominal pain

Anorexia

Diarrhea

Dyschesia

Dysphagia

Hematemesis

Hematochezia

Hypersalivation

Melena

Mucoid feces

Nausea

Regurgitation

Retching

Tenesmus

Vomiting

Weight loss

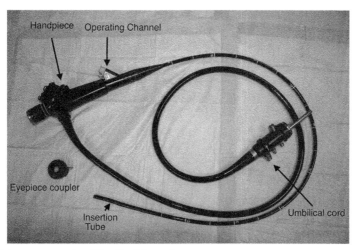

Fig. 1. Main components of the flexible endoscope.

to rinse the lens, and the working channel used for suction and endoscopic instruments. The tip of the endoscope can deflect in 4 directions under control of the 2 dials on the handpiece. Typically the degree of flexion is 90° in 3 planes and 180° in 1 plane (**Fig. 4**).

The umbilical cord connects the endoscope to support items including light source with insufflator, water, and suction (**Fig. 5**). Air, water, and vacuum are pumped through the umbilical cord for use through the insertion tube and are controlled with the hand-piece buttons. In a video endoscope, electronic signals are transmitted from the video chip in the endoscope to the external processor for image production on a monitor.

Support Items

A light source (xenon or halogen bulb) with insufflator, water bottle for flush, and suc-tion are used via the umbilical cord. Additional support items include a camera, cap-ture unit, and monitor (**Fig. 6**A). With a fiberoptic endoscope, a camera head can be

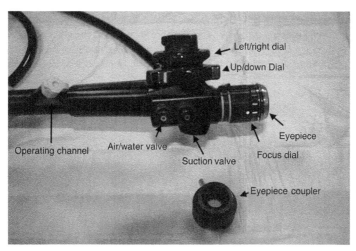

Fig. 2. Handpiece components of the flexible endoscope.

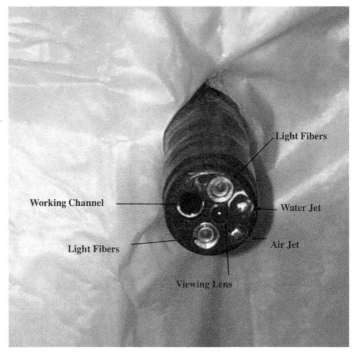

Fig. 3. End-on view of tip of insertion tube.

attached to the eyepiece and connected to an external camera for visualization on a monitor (see **Fig. 6**B). A video endoscope has a video microchip in the handpiece that sends electronic signals to a video processor that is included in the light source to produce an image on a monitor.

Endoscope Sizes

Endoscopes vary in diameter and length of the insertion tube (**Fig. 7**). When selecting an endoscope, the application of the scope should be considered. A longer insertion tube is necessary for giant breed dogs, whereas bronchoscopic examination in small dogs and cats will require a narrow insertion tube of 2.5 to 5 mm. Historically, it has been challenging to have 1 endoscope that adequately evaluates the gastrointestinal tract in all dogs and cats owing to the wide range of patient sizes. Bronchoscopy and

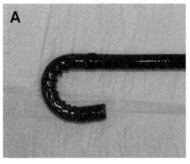
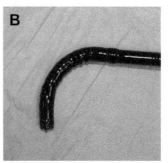

Fig. 4. (*A, B*) Flexion of tip of insertion tube.

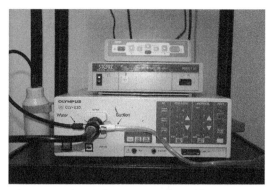

Fig. 5. Umbilical cord connected to light source and insufflator.

cystourethroscopy in the male dog place further demands on endoscope diversity. With advancement of flexible endoscopy, endoscopes with longer but narrower insertion tubes (7–9 mm diameter and 120–160 cm length) are available that also have adequate working channel size. A working channel that is large enough to pass a 2.4-mm (7-Fr) biopsy forceps or larger is recommended to obtain adequate tissue samples for histopathology.[2]

Endoscopic Instruments

Various instruments are available that pass through the working channel (**Fig. 8**). The most commonly used instruments for general gastrointestinal evaluation are biopsy forceps and grasping forceps for foreign body retrieval. A variety of styles are available. Additional instruments include cytology brushes and injection/aspiration needles. For advanced procedures and the experienced endoscopist, other instrumentation can be used via the working channel and are referenced in their respective sections elsewhere in this article.

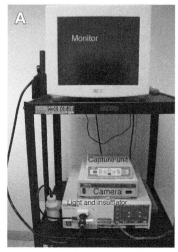
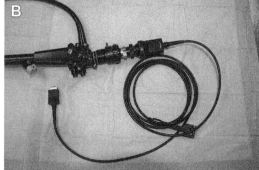

Fig. 6. (*A*) Endoscopic tower, including light source insufflator, camera, capture unit, and monitor. (*B*) Camera attachment for a fiberoptic endoscope.

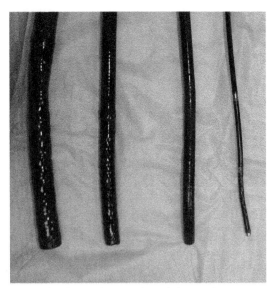

Fig. 7. Different diameter flexible endoscope from left to right: an 11-mm gastroduodeno-scope, an 8-mm gastroduodenoscope, a 5-mm bronchoscope, and a 2.5-mm urethroscope.

GENERAL FLEXIBLE ENDOSCOPY
Patient Preparation

Patients should be fasted for 12 hours before gastroduodenoscopy and 24 to 48 hours for colonoscopy, depending on the patient's condition and method of cleansing used. Isotonic electrolyte solutions such as GoLYTELY (Braintree Laboratories, Inc, Braintree, MA) will cause an osmotic diarrhea and typically provides adequate colon cleansing for endoscopic visualization. Failure to properly cleanse the colon impairs visibility and sample procurement.

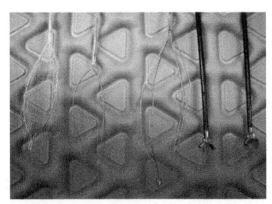

Fig. 8. Different foreign-body grasping devices: from left to right: basket, loop, wire basket, forceps with alligator jaws, and forceps with 1 × 2 teeth. (*From* Sum S, Ward CR. Flexible endoscopy in small animals. Vet Clin North Am Small Anim Pract 2009;39:886; with permission.)

Patient Positioning

For routine examination, the patient should be induced, intubated with a cuffed endo-tracheal tube to reduce the risk of aspiration, and maintained on inhalant anesthesia. The patient is placed in left lateral recumbency to minimize pressure on the stomach from adjacent organs and allow easier entry into the duodenum.

Approach

The endoscopist should be positioned in front of the head for gastroduodenoscopy and behind the tail for colonoscopy. If a monitor is used, it should be placed next to or behind the patient (**Fig. 9**). This positioning allows for direct visualization with coordination of the endoscope tip with the image on the screen. The placement of the monitor relative to the endoscopist is also important to minimize strain on the endoscopist, which can result in musculoskeletal discomfort such as tendinitis that can develop over time owing to compromised posture.

Procedure

Insufflation with air allows for distension and visualization of the lumen. The endoscope should only be advanced when the lumen is clearly visible. If visualization is not achieved or if orientation is lost, the insertion tube should be withdrawn slowly until the lumen is clearly visualized and then advanced. Contraction of the bowel may occur during the procedure, during which the endoscopist should pause until the stomach or intestinal musculature relaxes.

After visual evaluation is complete, tissue samples should be obtained from different areas for histopathology. The largest biopsy forceps that can pass through the operating channel should be used. The forceps can be advanced toward the site while trying to maintain a perpendicular approach to the mucosal wall. The forceps should be advanced firmly into tissue and, when resistance is met, the cups closed firmly. The biopsy forceps should be withdrawn with a steady tug from the mucosa. Deflating the

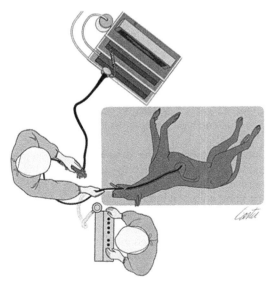

Fig. 9. Patient positioning for routine gastroduodenoscopy. (*From* Sum S, Ward CR. Flexible endoscopy in small animals. Vet Clin North Am Small Anim Pract 2009;39:889, with permission; and *Courtesy of* UGA, Athens, GA, 2009, with permission.)

lumen with suction can improve grasping of the mucosa. A minimum of 6 samples is recommended to ensure adequate quality; however, depending on sample size and location, additional samples may be necessary.[3]

Common procedures include esophagoscopy, gastroduodenoscopy, colonoscopy, and foreign body retrieval. Foreign body retrieval is typically limited to the esophagus and stomach. Treatment of esophageal strictures by dilation with balloon catheter is also a relatively simple procedure that is commonly performed in practice. These procedures have been described elsewhere.[1,4] Advanced flexible endoscopic procedures are currently being pursued more readily and show significant diagnostic and therapeutic potential.

STENT PLACEMENT FOR BENIGN OR MALIGNANT OBSTRUCTION

The use of stents in veterinary medicine has increased significantly. Although primarily used for tracheal and urogenital disorders such as tracheal collapse and bladder or prostate carcinoma, stents have been used in the gastrointestinal tract. Esophageal stenting in humans has been shown to be efficacious for esophageal obstruction.[5,6] However, complication rates are reported to be from 26% to 52%[7,8] and include tumor ingrowth in the mesh, overgrowth or granulation tissue at the stent margins, stent migration, bleeding, food impaction, esophageal injury, and chest pain. Types of stents used for esophageal stricture include biodegradable stents if short-term dilation is necessary, self-expanding plastic stents, and self-expanding metallic stents. The stents are available covered or uncovered. Nitinol stents have also been investigated and are available.[9]

Procedure

For veterinary patients, esophageal stent placement has been performed for benign and malignant esophageal obstruction. The procedure has been described in detail elsewhere.[9,10] Briefly, the patient is placed in lateral or dorsal recumbency depending on the placement of tacking sutures. Endoscopy is performed for identification and evaluation of the stricture, and partial balloon dilation performed to permit passage of the endoscope through the stricture to allow visualization of the caudal aspect of the lesion. A marker catheter is passed over an angle-tipped hydrophilic guidewire into the esophagus under fluoroscopic guidance and adjacent to the endoscope for radiographic measurement of the normal esophagus as well as the stricture. Stent diameter size is selected to be 10% to 20% larger than the normal esophagus caudal to the lesion. The length of the stent is selected such that 60% of the stent is cranial to the stricture when possible and extends past the thoracic inlet if tacking sutures are to be placed.

The constrained stent is passed over the guidewire alongside the endoscope under fluoroscopic guidance. It is passed through the stricture into the caudal esophagus. The stent is deployed such that 60% of the stent is cranial to the stricture. Esophageal patency and stent position are confirmed with endoscopy and fluoroscopy (**Fig. 10**). For tacking suture placement, the patient must be in dorsal recumbency and a 4- to 5-cm midline approach is performed before introduction of the stent, but with the endoscope in the esophagus. Blunt dissection to the cervical esophagus is performed until the endoscope can be palpated. When the appropriate area of the cervical esophagus is identified where the cranial aspect of the stent is expected, stent deployment can proceed. Two to 3 synthetic monofilament polypropylene sutures are placed to secure the stent to the cervical esophagus and the incision closed in standard fashion (**Fig. 11**).

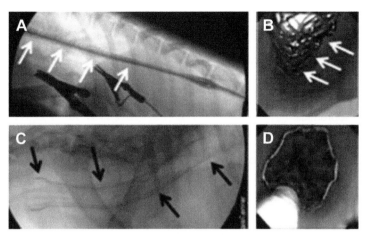

Fig. 10. (*A*) A constrained stent (*white arrows*) is passed across an intrathoracic esophageal stricture. (*B*) Endoscopic image obtained of the constrained stent (*white arrows*) before deployment. (*C*) Lateral fluoroscopic image after stent placement (*black arrows*) with the stent extending across the thoracic inlet for suture tacking if necessary. (*D*) Endoscopic image immediately after stent placement demonstrating good esophageal wall apposition. (*From* Lam N, Weisse C, Berent A, et al. Esophageal stenting for treatment of refractory benign esophageal strictures in dogs. J Vet Intern Med 2013;27:1066; with permission.)

Complications

- Ptyalism
- Regurgitation
- Gagging
- Nausea
- Megaesophagus
- Stent migration

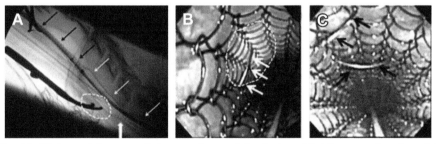

Fig. 11. (*A*) Lateral fluoroscopic image of a partially deployed (*white arrows*) and partial constrained (*black arrows*) esophageal stent. The Gelpi retractors are apparent at the caudal cervical surgical approach (*white dotted line*) where the suture tacking will take place. The stent is narrowed at the level of the stricture (*white block arrow*). (*B*) Endoscopic view showing a luminated area (*white dotted line*) where the operative approach has been made and the suture needle (*white arrows*) passing through the esophageal wall and engaging the stent. (*C*) Endoscopic view after 2 polypropylene sutures (*black arrows*) have been placed to tack the stent to the esophageal wall. (*From* Lam N, Weisse C, Berent A, et al. Esophageal stenting for treatment of refractory benign esophageal strictures in dogs. J Vet Intern Med 2013;27:1066; with permission.)

- Stent shortening
- Recurrence of esophageal stricture
- Hyperplastic ingrowth of tissue
- Tracheal–esophageal fistula

Postoperative Care

- H2 receptor antagonist or proton pump inhibitor
- Metoclopramide
- Antiemetics (maropitant citrate or ondansetron)
- Antibiotics if indicated
- Feed high-calorie gruel or canned food with gradual increase in consistency of diet

Outcomes

In the veterinary literature, several case reports describe the successful stent placement for management of esophageal stricture and neoplasia.[9,11,12] However, a retrospective study of 9 dogs with refractory benign esophageal stricture suggests a high risk of complications and poor long-term outcome with esophageal stenting in dogs.[10] Of the 9 dogs, 7 experienced complications resulting in additional procedures and only 3 of the 9 dogs received palliation of clinical signs beyond 6 months. Stricture recurrence or stent-related complications resulted in euthanasia in 4 dogs. Complications are listed in the previous section. Biodegradable stents tend to have a greater incidence of stricture recurrence and uncovered stents greater hyperplastic tissue ingrowth. A covered stent with tacking sutures is the current recommendation if an esophageal stent is considered.[10]

Limitations and Future Considerations

Stent placement for esophageal stricture is a relatively new procedure with limited information. The current literature has small patient numbers and variability in management among cases. There was also variation in stent type, location, or in additional security such as tacking sutures. In some patients, stent placement was a salvage procedure thereby creating selection bias. Although difficult, future evaluation ideally will control management and technique such that patient factors can be evaluated to determine ideal candidates and identify risk factors.

Colonic Stents

Colonic stent placement has been described in humans for treatment of benign and malignant obstructions. Technical and clinical success rates are reported to be high.[13–15] Complications reported include stent migration, colonic perforation, recurrent obstruction owing to tumor ingrowth, fistula formation, and tenesmus. Colonic stent placement has been reported in 1 dog and 2 cats with successful resolution of constipation.[16,17] All 3 patients were euthanized owing to disease-related complications, with 1 cat being euthanized 19 days after stent placement. Another cat and a dog survived for 274 and 238 days, respectively, after stent placement. The procedure described is similar to that for esophageal strictures (**Figs. 12** and **13**).

ENDOSCOPIC ULTRASONOGRAPHY AND ENDOSCOPIC ULTRASOUND-GUIDED FINE NEEDLE ASPIRATION OF THE PANCREAS
Endoscopic Ultrasonography

Endoscopic ultrasonography was introduced approximately 30 years ago in humans and has proven to be a reliable technique for assessing the abdominal cavity.[18–20]

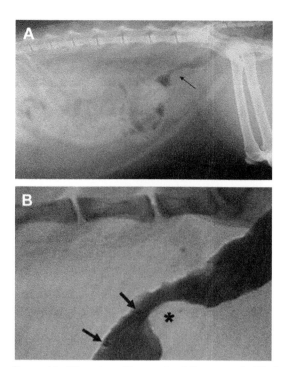

Fig. 12. Lateral radiographic (*A*) and positive-contrast fluoroscopic (*B*) views of a cat with intestinal adenocarcinoma causing colonic obstruction. (*A*) Notice the feces-filled ascending colon with a section of luminal narrowing (*arrow*) in the distal portion of the descending colon. (*B*) Notice the luminal stenosis (*asterisk*). A marking catheter with radiopaque markers (*arrows*) is positioned across the lesion. (*From* Hume DZ. Palliative use of a stent for colonic obstruction caused by adenocarcinoma in two cats. J Am Vet Med Assoc 2006;228:393; with permission.)

An ultrasound probe is mounted to a flexible endoscope[21] such that the endoscopist is able to evaluate both the lumen of hollow organs and the structures deep to the mucosa and adjacent organs (**Fig. 14**). The ultrasound probe has a closer proximity to deeper abdominal structures that permits the use of higher frequencies and minimizes compromise of the image owing to intestinal gas or fat.[19,21,22] The result is higher resolution images and improved identification of abdominal structures.

Procedure
Materials and methods for endoscopic ultrasound have been described elsewhere.[19–22] An ultrasound videogastroscope is supported by an ultrasound unit. The ultrasound endoscope contains a curved linear array transducer with a frequency range of 5 to 10 MHz. A nonsterile balloon that can be filled with water is placed over the insertion tube tip. The patient is prepared for routine gastroduodenoscopy or colonoscopy and placed in left lateral recumbency. Examination is similar to routine flexible endoscopy and several readily identifiable landmarks guide the examination. However, in human medicine 150 procedures are recommended for clinicians to learn the method and 250 to 500 to achieve clinical competency.[20] Readily identified structures include the portal vein and caudal vena cava, spleen, cranial duodenal flexure, left kidney, and aorta as the 5 primary landmarks. From the stomach, the liver,

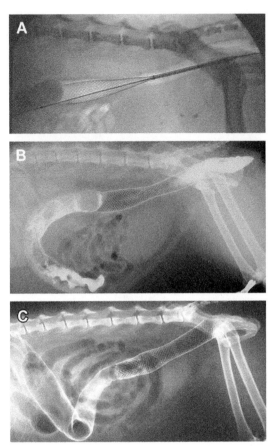

Fig. 13. Lateral abdominal radiographic views of a cat undergoing placement of a stent across a region of colonic obstruction caused by an adenocarcinoma. (*A*) Deployment of the stent across the lesion. (*B*) Twenty-four hours after stent placement. (*C*) Forty-eight hours after stent placement; notice alleviation of the colonic obstruction. (*From* Hume DZ. Palliative use of a stent for colonic obstruction caused by adenocarcinoma in two cats. J Am Vet Med Assoc 2006;228:393.)

gallbladder, bile ducts, kidneys, adrenal glands, body, and left limb of the pancreas can be visualized. Advancing the ultrasound endoscope into the duodenum allows for scanning of the right limb of the pancreas.[22]

Complications

- Difficulty passing endoscope ultrasound through the pylorus into the duodenum owing to the size and shape of the transducer with endoscope tip.
- Reduced flexibility of the tip of the endoscope owing to the ultrasound transducer.
- Limited visualization of abdominal structures owing to anatomic proximity to the stomach and duodenum.

Endoscopic Ultrasound-Guided Fine Needle Aspiration of the Pancreas

Procedure

Endoscopic ultrasound-guided fine needle aspiration of the pancreas is considered a safe procedure in humans. A recent experimental study in Beagles found it to be safe

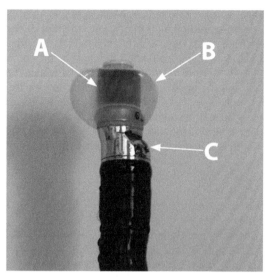

Fig. 14. The tip of the radial ultrasonographic gastrovideoscope used to perform endoscopic ultrasonography examinations in 14 anesthetized healthy Beagles in a study conducted to characterize the ultrasonographic appearance of the canine esophagus. Notice the red radial probe tip (A), the water-filled balloon that served as a standoff (B), and the optical device and working channel of the gastrovideoscope (C). The water-filled balloon provided a distance of approximately 2 mm between the probe tip and the esophageal wall. (*From* Baloi PA, Kircher PR, Kook PH. Endoscopic ultrasonographic evaluation of the esophagus in healthy dogs. Am J Vet Res 2013;74:1006; with permission.)

and feasible, although the entire pancreas can be difficult to visualize (**Fig. 15**).[22] The procedure for endoscopic-ultrasound guided fine needle aspiration is described. A 19-guage endoscopic ultrasound needle is used to aspirate the right limb of the pancreas with power Doppler imaging to avoid vasculature. A spiral metal sheath

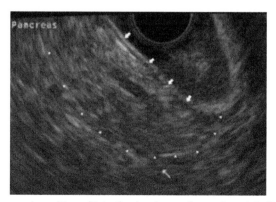

Fig. 15. The endoscope is positioned into the duodenum from where it is directed medially to visualize the pancreas, outlined with small white arrows. The pancreas is less homogeneous but delineated. It is landmarked by the vena pancreatic duodenale. (*From* Kook PH, Baloi P, Ruetten M, et al. Feasibility and safety of endoscopic ultrasound-guided fine needle aspiration of the pancreas in dogs. J Vet Intern Med 2012;26:515; with permission.)

connected to a biopsy handle supports the needle, and the apparatus is inserted into the biopsy channel and secured by a Luer-lock onto the biopsy channel. The needle and attached stylet is advanced under endoscopic and ultrasound guidance. The distance from the end of the needle sheath and the target is measured while the handle and adjustable needle stopper prevents the needle from advancing beyond the target. The stylet is retracted and the needle advanced forward by the thrust of the handle. When the tip of the needle is in the target, the stylet is removed and a 10-mL syringe is attached to apply negative pressure while the needle is moved within the target under ultrasound-guided control. Negative pressure is then released and the needle retracted into the sheath and locked. The needle assembly is removed and the cytologic samples made.

Complications

- Potential iatrogenic acute pancreatitis.
- Potential iatrogenic infection.
- Constraints on visualization. Sections of the pancreas that are not adjacent to the stomach or duodenum are not easily imaged.
- Technical strain with the ultrasound endoscope and complete needle device (sheath, biopsy needle, stylet, and handle) can be experienced. This strain affects maintenance of image of aspiration target.
- Immediate, on-site cytologic evaluation is ideal to minimize the risk of inadequate cellularity of the samples before recovery from anesthesia.
- The risks in the report were low with no complications; however, further evaluation in dogs with pancreatic disease is necessary.

Postoperative care

- Postoperative analgesia if indicated
- Monitoring for iatrogenic infection and pancreatitis
- Treatment as indicated for underlying disorder

Follow-up and clinical implications

Endoscopic ultrasonography can improve visibility of deeper abdominal structures and aid in the identification of lesions. Ultrasound-guided fine needle aspiration via endoscopy can improve diagnostic capability thereby providing better prognostic information and development of treatment plans.

Outcomes

The patients in this study experienced no adverse effects clinically and exhibited no laboratory abnormalities after the procedure.[22]

Limitations and future considerations

The pancreas can still be difficult to visualize with endoscopic ultrasonography. The skill and experience of the operator is a key factor in identifying abdominal structures and obtaining diagnostic samples. Further evaluation in patients with pancreatic disease is necessary.

ENDOSCOPIC RETROGRADE PANCREATOGRAPHY AND CHOLANGIOPANCREATOGRAPHY

Endoscopic retrograde pancreatography (ERP) and cholangiopancreatography (ERCP) use endoscopy and fluoroscopy to evaluate and image the biliary and pancreatic duct systems.[23] ERCP is used in humans for diagnosis of extrahepatic biliary problems and for the preoperative and postoperative management of patients undergoing gallbladder surgery. It is also used for cholelithiasis, stenting, or drainage of biliary and pancreatic ducts, and treatment of papillary stenosis with sphincterotomy or papillectomy via endoscopy. In humans, the common bile duct and pancreatic duct terminate together in the major papilla, making selective duct cannulation difficult.[24]

ERP and ERCP have been shown to be technically feasible in dogs. In contrast with humans, the common bile duct opens into the duodenum at the major papilla and the accessory pancreatic duct terminates in the minor papilla (**Fig. 16**).[25] Therefore, selective cannulation is possible to allow for endoscopic retrograde cholangiography or pancreatography as well as cholangiopancreatography.

Procedure

In contrast with standard gastroduodenoscopy, ERCP is performed in dorsal recumbency.[25] A side view flexible endoscope is required for ease of identification of the major and minor papillae as well as cannulation of the biliary and pancreatic ducts. A standard catheter used for ERCP is prefilled with iodinated contrast medium and passed through the working channel of the endoscope to insert into the papilla. There were 10 to 40 mL of contrast medium administered through the major papilla for cholangiography and 1.0 to 2.0 mL of contrast medium administered through the minor papilla for pancreatography. Contrast medium is injected under fluoroscopic guidance until the target area is filled (**Fig. 17**).

Complications

- Transient increase in serum pancreatic enzymes
- Difficulty cannulating pancreatic or biliary duct
- Potential for pancreatitis (reported in humans)
- Potential for hemorrhage (reported in humans)

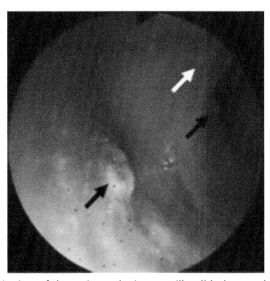

Fig. 16. Endoscopic view of the major and minor papillae (*black arrows*) and the accessory papilla (*white arrow*). (*From* Spillman T, Schnell-Kretschmer H, Dick M, et al. Endoscopic retrograde cholangio-pancreatography in healthy beagles. Vet Radiol Ultrasound 2005;46:99; with permission.)

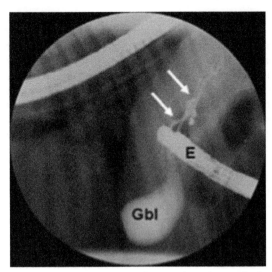

Fig. 17. Endoscopic retrograde cholangiography in a beagle. Marked structures are gall-bladder (Gbl), biliary ducts (*arrows*), and side view endoscope (E). (*From* Spillman T, Schnell-Kretschmer H, Dick M, et al. Endoscopic retrograde cholangio-pancreatography in healthy beagles. Vet Radiol Ultrasound 2005;46:100; with permission.)

- Potential for infection (reported in humans)
- Potential for perforation (reported in humans)

Postoperative Care

- As indicated for findings and clinical signs
- Ursodeoxycholic acid

Follow-up and Clinical Implications

Patients found to have filling defects may undergo medical therapy or surgical exploration. The nature of the filling defect can guide the clinician toward the appropriate therapeutic plan. Patients may be able to undergo minimally invasive treatment for biliary or pancreatic duct obstructions.

Outcomes

In 1 study of dogs with chronic gastrointestinal disease undergoing ERCP, 5 of 20 dogs had abnormal bile duct shape.[24] Two dogs had dilated bile ducts, 2 dogs had filling defects in the common bile duct, and 1 dog had a deviated position of the common bile duct suspicious for bile duct deformation. In the 2 patients with dilated bile duct and the 1 patient with suspected deformation, no further investigation was performed. In the remaining 2 patients, 1 was treated with oral ursodeoxycholic acid with successful resolution of clinical signs (**Fig. 18**). The other patient had minimal excretion of contrast medium after administration of ceruletide. ERC was repeated 5 days after the initial procedure with the same findings and papillar stenosis was diagnosed (**Fig. 19**). Clinical signs resolved after sphincterotomy was performed through the side view endoscope. A guidewire was placed via the ERCP catheter and the catheter removed. A sphincterotome was placed over the guidewire and pushed into the papilla. The papilla was cut electrosurgically.

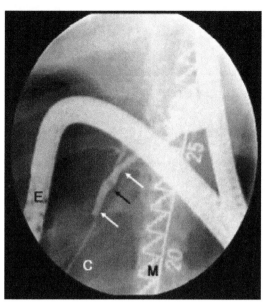

Fig. 18. Endoscopic retrograde cholangiography (dorsal recumbency) of a crossbreed (5 years old, female, 33 kg), with chronic recurrent abdominal pain for about 4 months: marked structures are endoscope (E), catheter (C), enlarged common bile duct (*white arrows*, maximum diameter 4.7 mm), and radiolucent filling defect (*black arrow*). M, radiopaque measure. (*From* Spillman T, Schnell-Kretschmer H, Dick M, et al. Endoscopic retrograde cholangio-pancreatography in dogs with chronic gastrointestinal problems. Vet Radiol Ultrasound 2005;46:293–99; with permission.)

ERP is the diagnostic tool of choice in humans to differentiate between inflammation and neoplasia.[22–25] Stages of pancreatitis can also be better assessed by this method. The utility of ERP in veterinary medicine could allow for better differentiation of the severity of pancreatic disease. Two patients in the study were diagnosed with end-stage pancreatic acinar atrophy and had alterations in the course of their left and right accessory pancreatic ducts compared with normal anatomy.[24] No clinical side effects were noted in dogs, although an increase in serum pancreatic enzyme levels (amylase or lipase) can be seen transiently in some dogs.

Cats are notoriously challenging for diagnosing and treating diseases of the gallbladder and pancreas. ERCP was evaluated recently in 4 healthy cats and found to be feasible, although technically challenging.[26] Identification of the major duodenal papilla was best accomplished using chromoendoscopy with 1 to 3 drops of undiluted 1% methylene blue through an ERCP catheter onto the duodenal mucosa. The presence of bile exiting the papilla was clearly visible with chromoendoscopy (**Fig. 20**). However, white light endoscopy failed to identify the major duodenal papilla in all cats. Cannulation of the duodenal papilla with an ERCP catheter was only possible in dorsal, and not in ventral, recumbency, similar to dogs and in contrast with humans. Complete ERCP was possible in 2 cats and ERP or ERC was achieved in the other 2. Because the pancreatic duct and common bile duct terminate in the major papilla and the feline papilla is smaller in size, an unselected filling with contrast occurs of the 2 duct systems based on placement of the ERCP catheter into the common junction of the 2 ducts versus inserting the catheter into the duct of 1 system (**Fig. 21**).

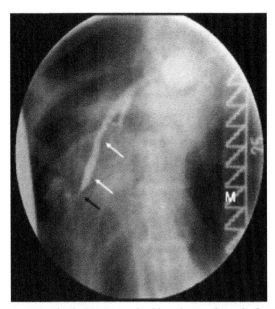

Fig. 19. Endoscopic retrograde cholangiography (dorsal recumbency) of a Great Munsterland (12 years old, male, 29 kg), with recurrent vomiting, diarrhea, and abdominal pain for about 9 months: marked structures are dilated common bile duct (*white arrows*, maximum diameter 4.5 mm) and stenotic papilla major during excretion of contrast medium into duodenum after stimulation of gallbladder contraction with ceruletide (*black arrow*). (*From* Spillman T, Schnell-Kretschmer H, Dick M, et al. Endoscopic retrograde cholangio-pancreatography in dogs with chronic gastrointestinal problems. Vet Radiol Ultrasound 2005;46:293–99; with permission.)

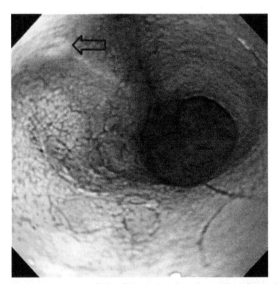

Fig. 20. Chromoendoscopic image of the feline duodenal papilla after administration of 2 to 3 drops of methylene blue. Note the yellow color that represents bile. The papilla (*arrow*) is the small slit in the mucosa. This image shows how difficult it could be to find the papilla if it was not highlighted by the dye. (*From* Spillman T, Willard MD, Ruhnke I, et al. Feasibility of endoscopic retrograde cholangiopancreatography in healthy cats. Vet Radiol Ultrasound 2014;55:87; with permission.)

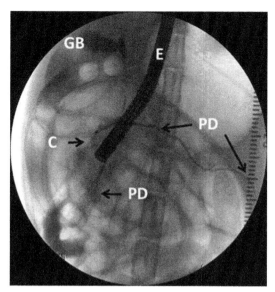

Fig. 21. Radiographic image acquired after endoscopic retrograde cholangiopancreatography in a cat. Notice that the endoscope (E) has been subjected to a shortening maneuver, that is, the duodenoscope has been straightened and adjusted to the angular fold with its tip in the proximal duodenum. C, catheter; GB, gallbladder; PD, pancreatic ducts. (*From* Spillman T, Willard MD, Ruhnke I, et al. Feasibility of endoscopic retrograde cholangiopancreatography in healthy cats. Vet Radiol Ultrasound 2014;55:87; with permission.)

No clinical side effects were observed with ERCP in the 4 cats in this study. Two cats had marked but temporary increases in feline pancreatic lipase immunoreactivity concentrations. Pancreatic biopsies were not obtained; therefore, a subclinical pancreatitis could not be ruled out. Similarly, ERCP causes transient increases in serum pancreatic enzyme levels.[23] Potential complications with ERCP include pancreatitis, hemorrhage, perforation, and infection. Overfilling of the gallbladder or pancreatic ducts resulting in contrast filling of the pancreatic parenchyma has been used to experimentally induce pancreatitis in dogs.[27] Additional limitations were encountered in performing ERCP. Dogs weighing less than 10 kg were unable to undergo ERCP because the diameter of the duodenum was too small for the side view endoscope. In addition, partial or total failure of performing ERCP occurred in 30% of dogs, usually owing to food remains or mucus obscuring the view of the papillae, difficulty in cannulation of the papillae, changes to the duodenal mucosa, and difficulty entering the pylorus of the stomach.[23]

Limitations and Future Considerations

ERCP can be challenging technically in small dogs and cats. However, the procedure can be performed safely and successfully. Further evaluation of ERCP in patients with biliary tract and pancreatic disorders is warranted.

NATURAL ORIFICE TRANSLUMINAL ENDOSCOPIC SURGERY

Natural orifice transluminal endoscopic surgery (NOTES) is an endoscopic procedure that allows access to the abdominal cavity without cutaneous incisions. NOTES is a relatively new procedure still under investigation in human medicine. Surgical access to the abdomen is achieved via the stomach, colon, or vagina.[28] Because of the method of access, it is hypothesized that the patient will experience less pain and disability with a quicker return to function. However, there is risk of bacterial contamination into the peritoneum. Instrument limitations exist, resulting in limited visibility of the operative field and occasionally impractical approaches to tissue manipulation for certain procedures.

Procedure

Recently, a veterinary feasibility study was conducted for oophorectomy in dogs.[29] Ten dogs underwent bilateral ovariectomy. The necessary equipment and procedure were described in detail. Patients are placed in dorsal recumbency and the abdomen clipped and prepared for aseptic surgery. The stomach is lavaged and then instilled with cefazolin (1 g/200 mL sterile 0.9% NaCl). A dual-channel endoscope is passed down to the stomach and transilluminates the ideal gastrotomy site. A guidewire is passed percutaneously into the stomach via an 18-guage catheter and pulled into the endoscope. A needle–knife is passed down to the stomach to create the gastrotomy.

An endoscopic balloon dilator is passed over the guidewire to dilate the gastrotomy. The endoscope is positioned behind the balloon and the 2 are passed together through the gastrotomy into the peritoneal cavity. Insufflation is achieved through the endoscope with room air. Alternatively, insufflation can be achieved percutaneously with a CO_2 laparoscopic insufflator. Once access to the peritoneal cavity is achieved, the endoscope is removed over the guidewire, leaving the wire in place for access to the abdominal cavity from the mouth. The endoscope is reintroduced into the abdominal cavity beside the guidewire.

The patient is tilted head down and to the right to improve visibility of the left ovary. An endoscopic electrocautery snare is passed through 1 working channel of the endoscope and endoscopic grasping forceps passed through the other channel. The forceps are passed through the loop of the snare to then grasp and elevate the ovary. The loop is positioned around the elevated ovary and when in position, the snare is activated to resect the ovary. The ovary is held with the grasping forceps or snare and removed with the endoscope. The right ovary is removed in a similar fashion (**Fig. 22**).

The gastrotomy site is closed with T-fasteners positioned at 12, 3, 6, and 9 o'clock positions (**Fig. 23**). A beveled cap is placed on the end of the insertion tube of the endoscope. The T-fastener has 2–0 nylon suture swaged to the center of a 1-cm hollow needle. The needle is loaded onto a delivery device to be passed through the working channel of the endoscope. Suction is applied to aspirate the gastric mucosa into the cap on the insertion tube. The needle is advanced into the tissue and the T-fastener deployed. Once the 4 T-fasteners are placed in their respective positions, the fasteners located across the incision from each other are secured with a closure element (12 o'clock and 6 o'clock; 3 o'clock and 9 o'clock). The stomach is deflated via the endoscope and the abdomen deflated via percutaneous catheter.

Complications

- Dropping an ovary into the abdominal cavity
- Incomplete excision of ovaries
- Ovarian bursa was mistaken for the ovary and the ovaries were not removed in 1 patient in heat
- Subcutaneous emphysema
- Potential for peritonitis
- Potential for infection

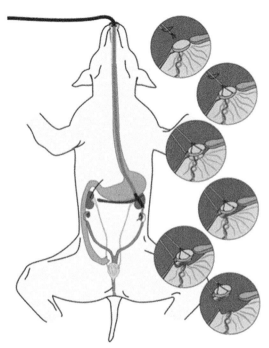

Fig. 22. The technique for performing natural orifice transluminal endoscopic surgery (NOTES) oophorectomy in dogs with a flexible therapeutic endoscope, snare, and 3-pronged grasping forceps. (*From* Freeman L, Rahmani EY, Sherman S, et al. Oophorectomy by natural orifice transluminal endoscopic surgery: feasibility study in dogs. Gastrointest Endosc 2009;69:1324; with permission.)

- Potential for hemorrhage.

Postoperative Care

- Analgesic (hydromorphone)
- Monitoring for pain and infection
- As indicated for procedure and clinical examination

Follow-up and Clinical Implications

Patients in the reported study were euthanatized at 10 to 14 days postoperatively.

Outcomes

Ten patients underwent oophorectomy. In the first 5 patients, 2 of the 5 patients had complete excision of both ovaries. Four of the 5 patients had complete excision of both ovaries in the second group. Two ovaries were dropped during the procedure for dogs in the first group.

Limitations and Future Considerations

Various limitations exist with NOTES. Currently, there is not an endoscopic instrument available that can cut and coagulate tissue. An electrocautery snare can be used; however, it is difficult to position with precision and it creates a wide zone of coagulation. The canine anatomy also provides the clinician with challenges because of the presence of the suspensory ligament, ovarian pedicle, and round ligament of

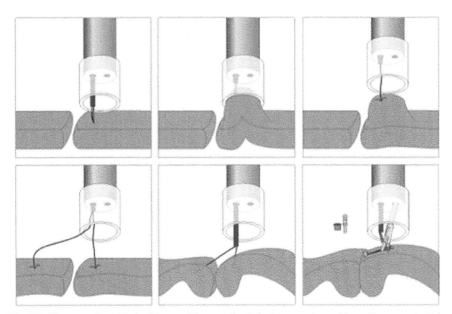

Fig. 23. Closure of gastric incisions with use of a T-fastener system. (*From* Freeman L, Rahmani EY, Sherman S, et al. Oophorectomy by natural orifice trasluminal endoscopic surgery: feasibility study in dogs. Gastrointest Endosc 2009;69:1325; with permission.)

the ovary. Adipose tissue is also typically present around the ovarian structures. Restrictions to access and visibility can lead to complications such as incomplete resection or failure to identify target structures.

NOTES was performed safely and somewhat effectively. Prospective evaluation in long-term surviving patients is necessary. NOTES is currently being investigated further in human medicine and may be used for other thoracic or abdominal procedures in veterinary medicine.

ENDOMICROSCOPY

Flexible endoscopy allows clinicians to assess in a minimally invasive manner a patient with gastrointestinal symptoms. Limitations with flexible endoscopy include the absolute number of samples to be obtained and delay in histopathology reporting. Confocal endomicroscopy uses flexible endoscopy in conjunction with microscopic imaging to provide immediate, histologically comparable imaging of the gastric and small intestinal mucosa. A miniature confocal microscope is integrated into a flexible endoscope to provide histologic detail of the mucosa. Alternatively, confocal miniprobes can be passed through the biopsy channel of a video endoscope. Fluorophores are administered to provide contrast for cellular detail in confocal images.[30,31]

Procedure

After routine white light endoscopy, exogenous fluorophores are administered. Fluorescein 10% aqueous solution is administered intravenously at 15 mg/kg intravenous bolus and/or acriflavine is applied topically to the mucosal surface via an endoscopic washing catheter. Confocal endomicroscopy is performed by placing the tip of the endoscope containing the microscope in a forward facing direction and in direct contact with the mucosal surface. Gentle suction stabilizes the image. Five sections, at a minimum, are evaluated per fluorophore. Intravenous administration of fluorescein provides 30 minutes of imaging and cellular cytoplasmic detail. With acriflavine, repeated application for visualization owing to elapsed time or to evaluate a new area may be necessary. Acriflavine provides subcellular, including nuclear, detail and therefore identification of individual cells (**Fig. 24**). It also allows for identification of *Helicobacter* and *Helicobacter*-like organisms.

Complications

- Visibility impaired owing to food and debris
- Image artifact owing to movement
- Reduced endoscope flexibility of endoscope insertion tube tip

Postoperative Care

- As indicated for disease

Follow-up, Clinical Implications, and Outcomes

The studies regarding endomicroscopy were in research colony animals and therefore follow-up and clinical implications were not evaluated in these reports. Because endomicroscopy is comparable with present-day gastroduodenoscopy, follow-up and clinical implications are similar owing to indications for pursuing gastroduodenoscopic

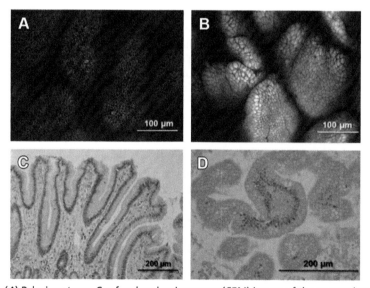

Fig. 24. (*A*) Pyloric antrum. Confocal endomicroscopy (CEM) image of the mucosal surface of the lower pyloric antrum. Only cellular cytoplasmic features are highlighted. Superficial imaging of the mucosal surface demonstrates the regular mosaic pattern of the epithelial cells. Image collected after intravenous administration of fluorescein. (*B*) Pyloric antrum. Topical administration of acriflavine results in preferential staining of nuclear contents providing superior visualization of individual cells and enhancing the superficial mosaic pattern. Histologic images of the pyloric antrum, including standard orientations (*C*) and orientations comparative with those obtained by using CEM (*D*) are also shown. (*From* Sharman MJ, Bacci B, Whittem T, et al. In vivo histologically equivalent evaluation of gastric mucosal topologic morphology in dogs by using confocal endomicroscopy. J Vet Intern Med 2014;28:801; with permission.)

evaluation. Diagnosis of conditions such as inflammatory bowel disease, *Helicobacter* gastritis, or neoplasia may be enhanced with confocal endomicroscopy.

Limitations and Future Considerations

Limitations with endomicroscopy are primarily related to the fact that imaging is a crucial part of the procedure. Food and debris obscure the image and therefore adequate fasting and patient preparation are necessary. Image artifact can also occur owing to motion or poor mucosal contact. Suction stabilizes contact of the endoscope to the mucosal surface. The flexibility of the endoscope is limited by the presence of the microscope in the tip of the insertion tube. Interpretation of confocal endomicroscopic images requires training and experience. Training that includes comparison of confocal endomicroscopic images to histopathology improves the investigator's ability to detect disease in vivo. There also seems to be a limitation to assessing deep mucosal and submucosal tissues. However, this has not been assessed in veterinary patients with gastrointestinal disease at this time. Adaptation of available technology may enable evaluation of deeper tissue structures.

Confocal endomicroscopy provides the advantage of better identification of superficial lesions and thereby focus endoscopic biopsies strategically to areas that may provide greater information. Other advantages of confocal endomicroscopy include the ability to evaluate a greater region and increased number of sites compared with histopathology samples because of the limitation in obtaining a number of biopsies.

In humans, confocal endomicroscopy has been used to identify a variety of gastrointestinal conditions, including dysplastic, neoplastic, inflammatory, and autoimmune diseases.[30,31] Identifiable microscopic changes are demonstrated in diseases including, but not limited to, atrophic gastritis, chronic inflammatory gastritis, intestinal metaplasia, and neoplastic diseases, such as tubular adenocarcinoma. Lesion identification during endomicroscopy helps to guide endoscopic biopsy and improves diagnostic yield. Future prospective evaluation of endomicroscopy in patients with clinical symptoms is warranted.

ENDOSCOPIC GASTROPEXY

Prophylactic gastropexy is often recommended in breeds that are recognized as predisposed to developing gastric dilatation volvulus (GDV). For various reasons, owners may elect to postpone or decline prophylactic gastropexy. A quicker, less invasive, and less expensive gastropexy procedure could increase client compliance and reduce the risk of GDV.

Procedure

An endoscopic gastropexy method was recently evaluated.[32] Patients were prepped for surgery in routine fashion after induction. Dogs were positioned in left oblique recumbency approximately 30° to the plane perpendicular to the operating table (**Fig. 25**). The gastroscope was passed orally to the stomach and the stomach insufflated until rugal folds were minimally visible. Identification of the gastropexy site was accomplished with external palpation across the body wall while visualizing the pyloric antrum. A stay suture was placed using size 0 or size 2 polypropylene suture on a cutting needle. The needle was passed through the right lateral aspect of the body wall immediately caudal to the 13th rib. The needle and suture were visualized in the pyloric antrum endoscopically as they entered and exited; the needle exited the body wall and the suture was pulled tight and secured with mosquito hemostats. An additional length of suture was passed 4 to 5 cm Aborad to the first suture position for a second stay

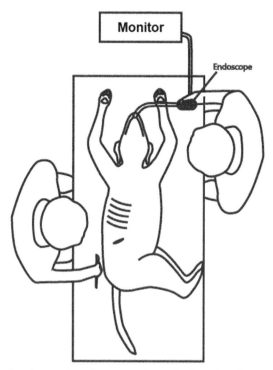

Fig. 25. Position of a dog undergoing an endoscopically assisted gastropexy. The dog is placed in left oblique recumbency at approximately 30° to a plane perpendicular to the operating table. One incision is made on the right side of the dog, just caudal to the 13th rib. (*From* Dujowich M, Reimer SB. Evaluation of an endoscopically assisted gastropexy technique in dogs. Am J Vet Res 2008;69:538; with permission.)

suture (**Fig. 26**). An incision was made between the 2 stay sutures parallel to the 13th rib through the layers of abdominal musculature until the stomach was visible. Gelpi retractors are used to improve visibility. A 3- to 4-cm longitudinal incision was made through the serosal and muscular layers of the pyloric antrum. The seromuscular layer was sutured to the transversus abdominus muscle in 2 individual continuous patterns. The obliquus externus abdominal muscles were apposed and sutured in a simple interrupted pattern followed by routine closure of the subcutaneous tissue and skin. The stay sutures were removed and the stomach decompressed with endoscopic visualization.

Complications

- Needle bending
- Needle breakage
- Hemorrhage
- Potential difficulty in approaching pyloric antrum for gastropexy owing to caudal ribs (not encountered)
- Potential for entrapment of loop of small intestine (not encountered)

Postoperative Care

The patients used in the study were euthanatized after the procedure for reasons unrelated to the study.

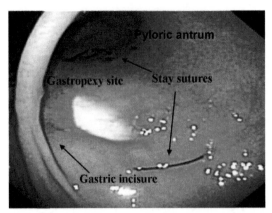

Fig. 26. Endoscopic view of the stomach of a dog undergoing endoscopically assisted gastropexy after stay sutures were placed in the pyloric antrum and the seromuscular layer was incised. The stay sutures are placed on the lateral portion of the abdomen just caudal to the 13th rib. (*From* Dujowich M, Reimer SB. Evaluation of an endoscopically assisted gastropexy technique in dogs. Am J Vet Res 2008;69:539; with permission.)

Follow-up, Clinical Implications, and Outcomes

Owing to the nature of the study, follow-up and outcome information is not available. However, no major complications were identified. The procedure was short and suspected to be relatively inexpensive. At necropsy, all gastropexy sites were determined to be sound with no damage to other abdominal organs nor entrapment of viscera.

Limitations and Future Considerations

Long-term results are not available for this procedure because all patients in the 1 study evaluating endoscopic gastropexy were euthanatized upon completion of the procedure. However, during the procedure, complications that occurred were limited to needle bending (5 instances in 2 dogs) and needle breakage (2 instances in 1 dog). The needle could not be retrieved in the second instance. Changing from size 0 polypropylene suture to size 2 polypropylene suture resolved the problem. Minor hemorrhage occurred with body wall incision and gastropexy procedure. Minimal blood was detected endoscopically with placement of the stay sutures. Post mortem physical inspection of the gastropexy site revealed proper position of the pexy and no complications.

Successful prophylactic gastropexy requires the formation of a permanent, strong adhesion without complications. Mesothelium between the serosal surface of the stomach and the body wall prevents the formation of an adhesion; therefore, the seromuscular layer of the stomach must be sutured to the transversus abdominus muscle. Correct anatomic position to prevent volvulus without interfering with normal gastric function is important to any gastropexy technique. Additionally, the procedure should have little to no complications and require minimal postoperative management of the patient. Endoscopic gastropexy may prove to be a reliable, inexpensive, and minimally invasive procedure to prevent GDV. Prospective long-term evaluation in animals at risk for GDV is warranted.

SUMMARY

As flexible endoscopy continues to gain popularity in veterinary medicine, its versatility should expand. Several novel minimally invasive diagnostic and therapeutic procedures are under investigation. Shorter recovery time and reduced morbidity are 2 major benefits of minimally invasive procedures. However, some of the techniques described herein should improve care for patients at risk for debilitating and life-threatening diseases and could have significant impact in small animal practice.

REFERENCES

1. Sum S, Ward CR. Flexible endoscopy in small animals. Vet Clin North Am Small Anim Pract 2009;39:881–902.
2. Goutal-Landry CM, Mansell J, Ryan KA, et al. Effect of endoscopic forceps on quality of duodenal mucosal biopsy in healthy dogs. J Vet Intern Med 2013;27: 456–61.
3. Willard MD, Mansell J, Fosgate GT, et al. Effect of sample quality on the sensitivity of endoscopic biopsy for detecting gastric and duodenal lesions in dogs and cats. J Vet Intern Med 2008;22:1084–9.
4. Tams TR, Rawlings CA. Small animal endoscopy. St Louis (MO): Elsevier; 2010.
5. Conio M, Repici A, Battaglia G, et al. A randomized prospective comparison of self-expandable metal stents in the palliation of malignant esophageal dysphagia. Am J Gastroenterol 2007;102:2667–77.
6. Selinger C, Ellul P, Smith P, et al. Oesophageal stent insertion for palliation of dysphagia in a district general hospital: experience from a case series of 137 patients. QJM 2008;101:545–8.
7. Freeman HJ. Endoscopic stenting – where are we now and where can we go? World J Gastroenterol 2008;14:3798–803.
8. Kim JH, Song HY, Shin JH, et al. Palliative treatment of unresectable esophogastric junction tumors: balloon dilation combined with chemotherapy and/or radiation therapy and metallic stent placement. J Vasc Interv Radiol 2008;19:912–7.
9. Hansen KS, Weisse C, Berent AC, et al. Use of a self-expanding metallic stent to palliate esophageal neoplastic obstruction in a dog. J Am Vet Med Assoc 2012; 240:1202–7.
10. Lam N, Weisse C, Berent AC, et al. Esophageal stenting for treatment of refractory benign esophageal strictures in dogs. J Vet Intern Med 2013;27:1064–70.
11. Battersby I, Doyle R. Use of a biodegradable self-expanding stent in the management of a benign oesophageal stricture in a cat. J Small Anim Pract 2010;51:49–52.
12. Glanemann B, Hildebrandt N, Schneider MA, et al. Recurrent single oesophageal stricture treated with a self-expanding stent in a cat. J Feline Med Surg 2008;10: 505–9.
13. Baron TH, Kozarek RA. Endoscopic stenting of colonic tumours. Best Pract Res Clin Gastroenterol 2004;18:209–29.
14. Khot UP, Lang AW, Murali K, et al. Systematic review of the efficacy and safety of colorectal stents. Br J Surg 2002;89:1096–102.
15. Watt AM, Faragher IG, Griffin TT, et al. Self-expanding metallic stents for relieving malignant colorectal obstruction. Ann Surg 2007;246:24–30.
16. Culp WTN, MacPhail CM, Perry JA, et al. Use of a nitinol stent to palliate a colorectal neoplastic obstruction in a dog. J Am Vet Med Assoc 2011;239:222–7.
17. Hume DZ, Solomon JA, Weisse CW. Palliative use of a stent for colonic obstruction caused by adenocarcinoma in two cats. J Am Vet Med Assoc 2006;228:392–6.
18. Zuccaro GJ, Sivak MVJ. Endoscopic ultrasonography in the diagnosis of chronic pancreatitis. Endoscopy 1992;24:347–9.
19. Morita Y, Mitsuyoshi T, Yasuda J, et al. Endoscopic ultrasonography of the pancreas in the dog. Vet Radiol Ultrasound 1998;39:552–6.

20. Gaschen L, Kircher P, Wolfram K. Endoscopic ultrasound of the canine abdomen. Vet Radiol Ultrasound 2007;48:338–49.
21. Baloi PA, Kircher PR, Kook PH. Endoscopic ultrasonographic evaluation of the esophagus in healthy dogs. Am J Vet Res 2013;74:1005–9.
22. Kook PH, Baloi P, Rueten M, et al. Feasibility and safety of endoscopic ultrasound-guided fine needle aspiration of the pancreas in dogs. J Vet Intern Med 2012;26:513–7.
23. Spillmann T, Happonen I, Sankari S, et al. Evaluation of serum values of pancreatic enzymes after endoscopic retrograde pancreatography in dogs. Am J Vet Res 2014;65:616–9.
24. Spillman T, Schnell-Kretschmer H, Dick M, et al. Endoscopic retrograde cholangio-pancreatography in dogs with chronic gastrointestinal problems. Vet Radiol Ultrasound 2005;46:293–9.
25. Spillmann T, Happonen I, Kahkonen T, et al. Endoscopic retrograde cholangio-pancreatography in healthy beagles. Vet Radiol Ultrasound 2005;46:97–104.
26. Spillman T, Willard MD, Ruhnke I, et al. Feasibility of endoscopic retrograde cholangiopancreatography in healthy cats. Vet Radiol Ultrasound 2014;55:85–91.
27. Ruben SD, Scorpio DG, Buscaglia JM. Refinement of canine pancreatitis model: inducing pancreatitis by using endoscopic retrograde cholangiopancreatography. Comp Med 2009;59:78–82.
28. Freeman L, Rahmani EY, Burgess RCF, et al. Evaluation of the learning curve for natural orifice transluminal endoscopic surgery: bilateral ovariectomy in dogs. Vet Surg 2011;40:140–50.
29. Freeman LJ, Rahmani EY, Sherman S, et al. Oophorectomy by natural orifice transluminal endoscopic surgery: feasibility study in dogs. Gastrointest Endosc 2009;69:1321–32.
30. Sharman MJ, Bacci B, Whittem T, et al. In vivo confocal endomicroscopy of small intestinal mucosal morphology in dogs. J Vet Intern Med 2013;27:1372–8.
31. Sharman MJ, Bacci B, Whittem T, et al. In vivo histologically equivalent evaluation of gastric mucosal topologic morphology in dogs by using confocal endomicroscopy. J Vet Intern Med 2014;28:799–808.
32. Dujowich M, Reimer SB. Evaluation of an endoscopically assisted gastropexy technique in dogs. Am J Vet Res 2008;69:537–41.

Advances in Urinary Tract Endoscopy

Allyson C. Berent, DVM

KEYWORDS

- Endourology • Endoscopy • Ureteral stenting • Endoscopic nephrolithotomy
- Sclerotherapy for idiopathic renal hematuria • Ureteroscopy
- Percutaneous cystolithotomy (PCCL) • Lithotripsy

KEY POINTS

- Endoscopic-assisted diagnostic and treatment options for urologic disease are becoming the standard of care in veterinary medicine.
- Ureteral obstructions should be considered an emergency and decompression can be performed endoscopically in dogs using ureteral stents, a procedure that holds the lowest morbidity and mortality.
- The combination of endoscopy and fluoroscopy allows for the diagnosis and treatment of various upper urinary tract diseases like ureteral stenting, endoscopic nephrolithotomy, laser ablation of ectopic ureters, sclerotherapy, or ureteroscopy/electrocautery for renal hematuria.
- Proper training and expertise in these endourologic techniques should be acquired before performing them on clinical patients for the best possible outcomes.

Interventional endoscopy uses endoscopy with or without fluoroscopy or ultrasonography to gain access to various parts of the body for various diagnostic and therapeutic endeavors. The most common organ system in veterinary medicine that uses this technology for visualization is the urinary tract. Over the past decade, these therapeutic and diagnostic modalities have become increasingly more accessible to veterinary patients,[1–17] similar to the experience in human medicine.

There are many advantages to using urinary tract endoscopic techniques, particularly compared with traditional surgical alternatives. Aside from reduced morbidity and mortality, image-guided therapies allow new treatment options for many conditions for which traditional surgery was either not possible, contraindicated, or met with severe complications.

With the high incidence of upper and lower urinary tract disease and the invasiveness and morbidity associated with traditional techniques, endourology has become

Dr A.C. Berent is a consultant for both Norfolk Vet Products and Infiniti Medical, which distribute various medical devices that are discussed in this article.
Interventional Endoscopy Services, Department of Small Animal Internal Medicine, The Animal Medical Center, 510 East 62nd Street, New York, NY 10065, USA
E-mail address: Allyson.Berent@amcny.org

Vet Clin Small Anim 46 (2016) 113–135
http://dx.doi.org/10.1016/j.cvsm.2015.07.003
0195-5616/16/$ – see front matter © 2016 Elsevier Inc. All rights reserved.

appealing in the practice of veterinary medicine. In this article, some of the most common urologic endoscopy procedures being performed in small animal veterinary patients are reviewed.

KIDNEY
Endoscopic Approach to Nephrolithiasis

Nephrolith removal is rarely necessary in veterinary medicine and should be considered only when the stones are problematic: causing intractable pyelonephritis despite appropriate medical management/dissolution when indicated; causing a ureteral outflow tract obstruction associated with hydronephrosis; or enlarging and overtaking the renal parenchyma, resulting in progressive renal damage. Most nephroliths do not seem to cause pain or discomfort unless they are associated with pyelonephritis, pyonephrosis, or a ureteral outflow obstruction, so the need for removal is rarely necessary. There is some concern that dogs with progressive renal insufficiency may benefit from stone removal, but this is not clinically proved.

Surgical options to treat nephroliths include nephrotomy, pyelotomy, and ureteronephrectomy and are reported to be associated with frequent complications and high long-term morbidity. In 1 study,[18] 43% of dogs had stone fragments remaining after surgery, a 23% complication rate was associated with the procedure, and 67% of dogs developed renal azotemia postoperatively. In a study of normal cats in which a nephrotomy was performed,[19] there was a 10% to 20% decrease in the glomerular filtration rate (GFR) after the surgery. In clinical patients, with previous renal injury associated with the uroliths, compensatory mechanisms are often exhausted before the diagnosis, implying that similar surgical interventions would have a more detrimental effect on renal function. In addition, knowing that more than 30% of adult cats develop renal azotemia, losing 10% to 20% of function from a nephrotomy can be a life-threatening procedure. In the author's opinion, open surgical nephrotomy should always be avoided whenever possible, and other options such as extracorporeal shock-wave lithotripsy (ESWL) or endoscopic nephrolithotomy (ENL) should be considered.

Extracorporeal shock-wave lithotripsy

ESWL refers to the fragmentation of stones using external shock waves that pass through a water bag, through the soft tissues of the patient, and are directed onto the stone using fluoroscopic guidance. The stone(s) is shocked at different energy levels based on location and stone composition, to facilitate it breaking up into small fragments that are able to pass down the ureter and into the urinary bladder over a 2-week to 12-week period.

ESWL is typically reserved for nephroliths and ureteroliths in dogs and is not recommended in cats[3–5,20] because of their type of stone (calcium oxalate monohydrate), which is resistant to fragmentation,[21] and the small size of their ureteral lumen (0.3 mm), making stone fragments unlikely to pass successfully. ESWL is believed to be safe for the canine kidney, although subclinical intrarenal hemorrhage does occur.[3–5] Studies have shown minimal effect of ESWL on GFR in both the short-term and long-term.[22,23] The availability of ESWL for veterinary patients is limited and is routinely available only at Purdue University (Dr Larry Adams) and the Animal Medical Center, New York (Dr Allyson Berent).

In dogs, ESWL fragmentation is successful, but up to 30% of dogs require more than 1 treatment to achieve adequate fragmentation of nephroliths.[3–5] Mortality with ESWL is less than 1%, with the most common complication being the development of a transient ureteral obstruction in approximately 10% of cases.[3–5] The risk of ureteral obstruction may be minimized by placement of a ureteral stent concurrently (see later discussion) before ESWL treatment to allow for passive ureteral dilation and prevent obstruction during fragment passage[24] (**Fig. 1**). Ureteral stent placement is typically performed endoscopically through the ureterovesicular junction (UVJ) before ESWL. For stones larger than 1.5 cm, ENL is often recommended in both human and veterinary patients (see later discussion).

Endoscopic nephrolithotomy

ENL (**Fig. 2**) can be performed either percutaneously (percutaneous nephrolithotomy [PCNL]) or under surgical assistance (surgically assisted ENL [SENL]) and is reserved for problematic nephroliths larger than 1.5 cm, or of cystine composition, which are notoriously resistant to ESWL.

This procedure has been shown to have minimal ill effect on renal function in humans[25] and is reported to be highly renal sparing compared with the alternatives because of the lack of nephron transection, because parenchymal dilation and spreading are used, which spares functional renal tissue.[22,25,26]

PCNL/SENL was recently reported in abstract form in 9 dogs and 1 cat.[7] The success rate of PCNL has been documented at 90% to 100% in both the adult and pediatric human populations, and the author has experienced the same in veterinary patients. Proper training and appropriate equipment are needed for a successful outcome.

Idiopathic renal hematuria

Essential (idiopathic) renal hematuria (IRH) is a rare condition, typically seen in young large-breed/giant-breed dogs, in which a focal area of bleeding in the upper urinary tract results in severe, often chronic, hematuria. This situation leads to the potential for iron deficiency anemia and blood clot formation, which can result in a ureteral or urethral obstruction. This condition is documented to occur bilaterally in 25% to 33% of affected dogs. The upper tract bleeding should be confirmed by cystoscopic evaluation of the UVJ and a jet of bloody urine is visualized (**Fig. 3**). Traditionally, a ureteronephrectomy was recommended to treat this condition, but this approach should be considered contraindicated because of the risk of progressive bilateral disease, the benign nature of the condition, the lack of disease of the functional renal tissue, and the availability and ease of newer kidney-sparing techniques.

In people, a hemangioma, angioma, or vascular malformation are the most common causes and are typically treated with ureteronephroscopy using electrocautery.[27,28] In veterinary patients, this treatment is often not possible because of their small ureter and lack of available equipment.

Sclerotherapy

Sclerotherapy can be performed using sterile liquid silver nitrate and povidone-iodine as cauterizing agents that are infused into the renal pelvis. Sclerotherapy can be performed in any dog (male or female), regardless of size. Under cystoscopic and fluoroscopic guidance, the cauterizing agent is infused into the renal pelvis through a ureteral occlusion balloon catheter (see **Fig. 3**). In a recent study,[8] sclerotherapy was used for the treatment of IRH and complete cessation of macroscopic hematuria occurred in 4 of 6 dogs within a median of 6 hours (range, postoperative to 7 days). Two additional dogs improved, 1 moderately and 1 substantially. None of the dogs required nephrectomy. The author has performed this procedure in more than 20 dogs, with success rates exceeding 80%.

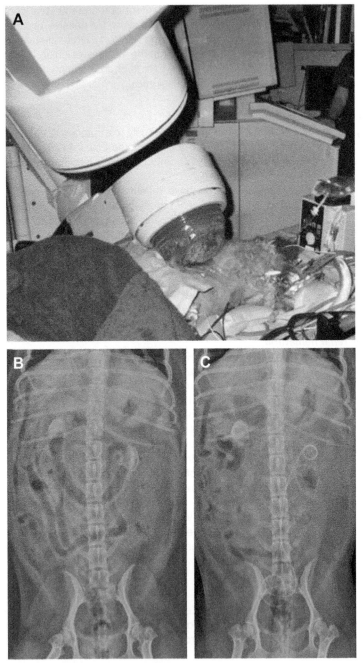

Fig. 1. EWSL in a female shih tzu for bilateral nephroliths. (*A*) Patient on the fluoroscopy table with the lithotrite water bag against the kidney and the fluoroscopy unit aligned to visualize the kidney stone. (*B*) Ventrodorsal radiograph of the dog before left-sided ESWL and ureteral stent placement. (*C*) Ventrodorsal radiograph immediately after ESWL and endoscopic ureteral stent placement.

Ureteroscopy
Ureteroscopy for electrocautery has been performed in only a few patients and is typically reserved for those that have failed sclerotherapy and have a large enough ureter to accept the 8-Fr ureteroscope (see **Fig. 3**). No complications were noted from the procedure when a stent was placed after infusion. Dogs need to be larger than approximately 20 kg for naive ureteroscopy, and approximately 8 to 10 kg if a ureteral stent is preplaced 10 to 14 days before the ureteroscopy. With preplacement of a ureteral stent, passive ureteral dilation occurs, allowing the passage of the ureteroscope.

URETERAL INTERVENTIONS

Ureteral obstructions have been seen more commonly in veterinary medicine in the past decade and are a concerning dilemma for patients. The invasiveness and morbidity/mortality associated with traditional surgical techniques[29–31] make the use of endourologic alternatives appealing.

The physiologic response to a ureteral obstruction results in a rapid decrease in GFR and severe progressive renal damage,[32,33] necessitating timely decompression for the best outcome. The composition of most ureteroliths in dogs (~50%) and cats (>95%) is calcium based, making dissolution completely contraindicated in cats and it should not be considered in dogs without concurrent decompression.[2,9–11,29,30,34–36] With medical management being effective in a few feline patients (8%–13%)[29] and traditional surgical interventions being associated with a relatively high perioperative complication (31% in cats and ~7%–15% in dogs)[29–31] and mortality (18%–21% in cats and 6.25% in dogs),[29–31] medical therapy should be considered when possible for 24 to 48 hours. Endoscopic alternatives, like ureteral stenting, are shown to result in immediate decompression, long-term obstruction relief, fewer perioperative complications than surgical alternatives, lower perioperative mortality, successful treatment of all causes of obstruction (stone, stricture, tumor), and a decreased recurrence rate of future obstructions.[9–11,34–36]

Benign Ureteral Obstruction

Traditional ureteral surgery
Traditional ureteral surgery for obstructive ureterolithiasis includes ureterotomy, neo-ureterocystostomy, ureteronephrectomy, or renal transplantation.[29–31] In a small study in dogs,[31] results after a ureterotomy, pyelotomy, or ureteronephrectomy were associated with surgical mortality of 6.25%, with 15% requiring additional surgery for reobstruction within 30 days. In addition, 43% of dogs in this study had evidence of recurrent urinary tract infections after surgery, 21% remained azotemic, and 15% had worsening azotemia. In cats, the procedure-associated complication and mortality are reported to be 30% and 21%, respectively. Most complications associated with surgery are caused by ureterotomy site edema, nephroliths that pass from the renal pelvis to the surgical site, stricture formation, missed ureteroliths, and surgery-associated urine leakage.[29,30]

Subcutaneous ureteral bypass device in cats
A subcutaneous ureteral bypass (SUB) device in cats is considered the treatment of choice in cats with ureteral obstructions because of the lowest reported morbidity and mortality compared with other options for feline decompression. Because this procedure is performed interventionally with fluoroscopic and surgical assistance and is not performed endoscopically,[35] it is not expanded on in this article. Instead, the reader is referred to other sources.[21,34–36]

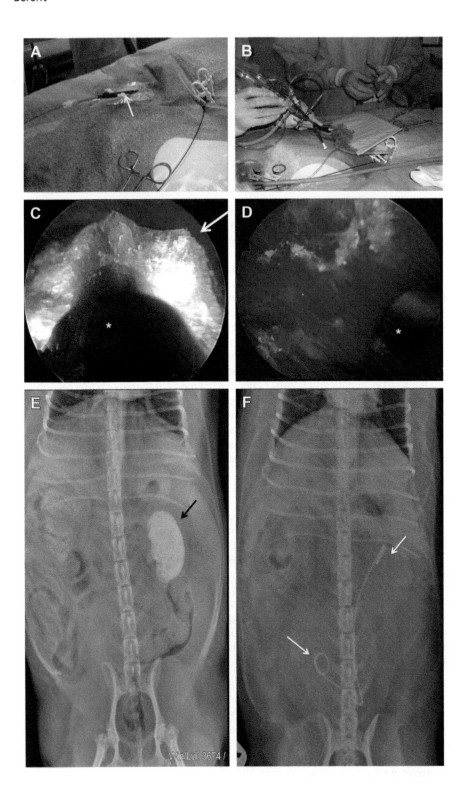

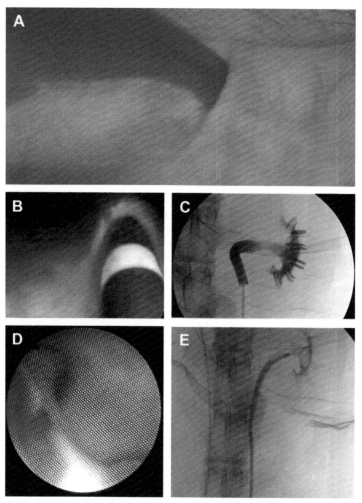

Fig. 3. Left-sided IRH in a female dog. (*A*) Endoscopic image with dog in dorsal recumbency showing a jet of hemorrhagic urine from the left UVJ. (*B*) An open-ended ureteral catheter up the left UVJ. (*C*) A ureteropelvic junction balloon up the ureter and a contrast study showing the filling of the renal pelvis during sclerotherapy. (*D*) A nephroscopic image during ureteronephroscopy showing a bleeding lesion. (*E*) Fluoroscopic image of the ureteroscope entering the renal pelvis of a dog with IRH.

Fig. 2. PCNL in a dog with a large left nephrolith. (*A*) Sheath (*yellow arrow*) inside the renal pelvis with a guide wire passed through the sheath, down the ureter, into the bladder, and out the urethra. (*B*) Endoscope inside the renal pelvis for lithotripsy. (*C*) Lithotrite (*white asterisk*) through the working channel of the endoscope breaking up the large nephrolith (*white arrow*). (*D*) Nephroscopy after the stone has been removed (*white asterisk is lithotrite*). (*E*) Ventrodorsal radiograph of the dog before PCNL showing the large nephrolith (*black arrow*). (*F*) Double pigtail ureteral stent (*white arrows*) in place after PCNL showing removal of the entire nephrolith.

Ureteral stents

Ureteral stents are used in humans to divert urine from the renal pelvis into the urinary bladder for obstructions secondary to ureterolithiasis, ureteral stenosis/strictures, malignant neoplasia, or trauma.[37–41] The main type of ureteral stents used in both human and veterinary patients is an indwelling double pigtail ureteral stent (**Fig. 4**). The double pigtail stent is completely intracorporeal and is 2.5 Fr in diameter in feline patients and 3.7, 4.7, or 6 Fr in canine patients. In human medicine, it is recommended that the stents be removed or exchanged after 3 to 6 months,[38,41,42] but this does not seem to be necessary in feline or canine patients because they have remained patent and in place for more than 6 years in some patients. Stent placement may be considered a long-term treatment option for various causes of ureteral obstructions; however, there may be potential side effects and long-term complications.[2,21,34,36,43]

Feline ureteral stents

Feline ureteral stents are typically placed under surgical assistance and only 10% to 15% are successfully placed endoscopically (**Fig. 5**). In a recent study in 69 cats (79 ureters),[34] that had ureteral stents placed either endoscopically or with surgical assistance, the cause of the ureteral obstruction was either stones (~75%) or strictures (~25%). After the stent was placed, 95% of patients had significant improvement in their azotemia and there was perioperative mortality of 7.5%; none of the patients died of stent placement complications or a persistent/recurrent ureteral

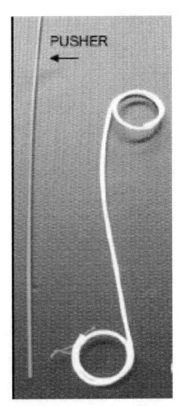

Fig. 4. Double pigtail ureteral stent with a pushing catheter used for the endoscopic treatment of ureteral obstructions.

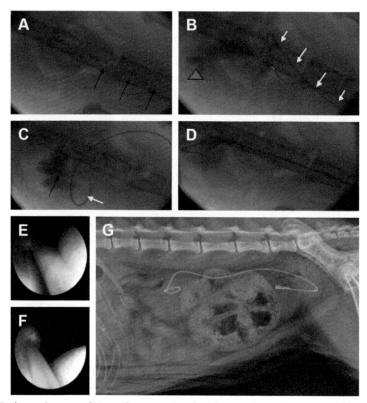

Fig. 5. Endoscopic ureteral stent placement in a female cat using endoscopic and fluoroscopic guidance. (*A*) Fluoroscopic image of a patient in dorsal recumbency. Guide wire (*black arrows*) being advanced up the ureter from the UVJ. (*B*) Open-ended ureteral catheter (*yellow arrows*) being advanced over the guide wire to a stone (*red arrow*) and a retrograde ureteropyelo-gram performed showing hydronephrosis (*red arrowhead*) and hydroureter. (*C*) Guide wire (*black arrow*) readvanced through the catheter (*yellow arrow*), around the stones, and into the renal pelvis. (*D*) Stent being advanced over the guide wire and being coiled inside the renal pelvis. (*E*) Endoscopic image of the guide wire being advanced into the right UVJ. (*F*) Ureteral catheter being advanced over the guide wire visualized using cystoscopy. (*G*) Lateral radiograph of the cat after the ureteral stent is in place with 1 pigtail in the urinary bladder and the other in the renal pelvis.

obstruction.[9] The most common poststent complication seen in cats was dysuria (≤38%) and reocclusion (~25%) requiring stent exchange or the use of a SUB device.[1,2,21,35,36]

Canine Ureteral Stenting for Benign Disease

The use of double pigtail ureteral stents (**Fig. 6**) in dogs has been investigated as an alternative to traditional surgery, resulting in immediate ureteral decompression, sta-bilization of the associated azotemia, a decreased risk of ureteral stricture or ureteral leakage, and a decreased rate of ureteral obstruction recurrence.[9–11] Ureteral stents in dogs, when placed for stone-induced or stricture-induced obstructions, are typically placed endoscopically, with high success rates (>90%).[9–11] The most common com-plications with canine ureteral stents are recurrent urinary tract infections (15%–59%), stent occlusion (<10%), migration (6%), encrustation (<5%), and proliferative tissue at

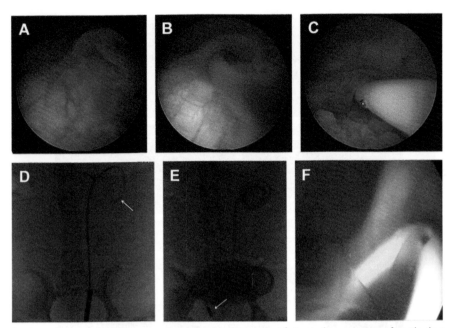

Fig. 6. Endoscopic and fluoroscopic images during ureteral stent placement in a female dog. The patient is in dorsal recumbency. (*A*) Left UVJ visualized with the cystoscope. (*B*) Guide wire being advanced up the UVJ. (*C*) Open-ended ureteral catheter being advanced over the guide wire. (*D*) Fluoroscopic image of the wire (*white arrow*) and catheter (*black arrow*) advanced to the renal pelvis. (*E*) Double pigtail ureteral stent (*blue arrow*) being deployed and pushed into the urinary bladder (*yellow arrow*) with a pusher catheter. (*F*) Endoscopic image once the stent is deployed in the bladder and urine is seen coming from the side holes of the stent.

the UVJ. These issues are not usually life threatening and are typically easy to address on an outpatient basis.

In dogs, ureteral stenting is almost always performed endoscopically using fluoroscopic guidance by gaining access cystoscopically to the ureter through the UVJ. Once the renal pelvis is catheterized, it is drained and lavaged, especially if this is associated with a pyonephrosis.[10] Then, the appropriately sized ureteral stent is placed over the guide wire through the working channel of the cystoscope using fluoroscopic guidance. The patient is typically discharged the same day as the procedure.

This procedure has been successful minimally invasively in more than 90% of dogs, and the reported mortality was less than 2%.[10,11] Recurrent urinary tract infection (15%–59% after stent vs ~60%–80% before stent)[10,11] was also reported after traditional surgery, making it unlikely to be associated with the presence of the stent but rather with the concurrent stone disease, established pyelonephritis, decreased renal function, concurrent urethral incompetence, and concurrent immune dysfunction of the patient. When a ureteral stent is removed because of complete stone dissolution, in the case of struvite ureterolithiasis, chronic infections can still be seen months and years after stent removal. Careful monitoring of image findings, urinalysis, and cultures are required to avoid ascending pyelonephritis. Cystoscopic-assisted ureteral stent placement is technically challenging and should not be attempted without proper endourology training. For canine patients suspected of having struvite ureterolithiasis, successful dissolution after ureteral stent placement is documented with a dissolution diet and long-term antibiotics. This strategy should always be adopted and cases carefully followed up when struvite stones are present or suspected (A.C. Berent, Direct communication, 2015).

Canine malignant ureteral obstruction

Canine malignant ureteral obstruction associated with trigonal obstructive neoplasia is typically performed using both ultrasonography and fluoroscopic guidance and is rarely possible endoscopically. For cases in which prophylactic ureteral stents are desired, this technique can be performed endoscopically, before ureteral occlusion from the trigonal tumor, while the UVJ is still endoscopically visible (**Fig. 7**).

Cystoscopic-guided laser ablation of ectopic ureters

Cystoscopic-guided laser ablation of ectopic ureters (CLA-EU) is a minimally invasive treatment option for intramural ectopic ureters. More than 95% of ectopic ureters traverse intramurally and exit into the urethra, making endoscopic repair a treatment for most patients.[44]

Endoscopic repair of ectopic ureters has been performed over the past 8 to 10 years in both male and female dogs using a combination of fluoroscopy, cystoscopy, and a diode or holmium: YAG laser[13–15] (**Figs. 8** and **9**). The laser is used to transect the medial aspect of the ureteral wall, separating the ectopic ureter from the normal trigone and urethra. This procedure can be performed on an outpatient basis, usually at the time of diagnosis, avoiding the need for less sensitive diagnostic tools, like ultrasonography and computed tomography. During the CLA-EU procedure, various vaginal anomalies can be concurrently treated with laser therapy (see later discussion).

After CLA-EU, the ureteral orifice has been shown to remain in a normal position at the trigone of the bladder, but many dogs have concurrent urethral incompetence[13] and require additional medication or procedures to maintain continence.[45] A prospective study of CLA-EU in 30 female dogs reported an overall urinary continence rate of 77% after CLA-EU with the addition of medical management, collagen injections, or placement of a urethral hydraulic occluder.[13,46] After laser ablation in male dogs, the continence rate has been reported in a small group of dogs to be 100%,[15] and in the author's experience, in a larger group of dogs it remains approximately 85% (A.C. Berent, Direct communication, 2015). The success rate of the CLA-EU procedure alone in female and male dogs is approximately 56%. The addition of a hydraulic occluder has been reported to increase the continence rate to 92%.[46]

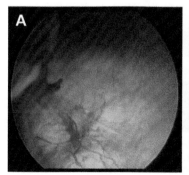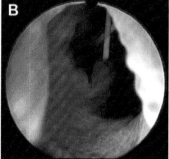

Fig. 7. Endoscopic images of a female dog with trigone transitional cell carcinoma. Patient is in dorsal recumbency. (*A*) Tumor approaching the opening of the right UVJ. (*B*) Stent in the ureter exiting the UVJ among a tuft of tumor at the trigone.

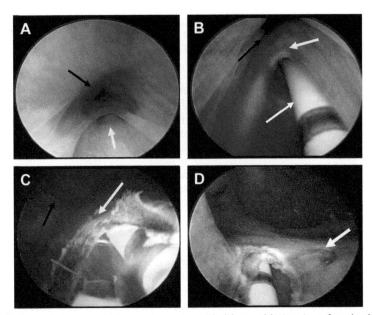

Fig. 8. Endoscopic images during cystoscopic-guided laser ablation in a female dog of a right unilateral intramural ectopic ureter. Patient is in dorsal recumbency. (*A*) Urethral image showing the ectopic ureteral opening (*yellow arrow*) within the urethra (*black arrow*). (*B*) Open-ended ureteral catheter (*white arrow*) cannulating the ureteral opening (*yellow arrow*) and advanced up the ureter (*black arrow*) to show the path of the ectopia. (*C*) A diode laser (*red arrow*) cutting the ectopic tissue next to the catheter while advancing the ectopic ureteral opening (*yellow arrow*) toward the trigone (*black arrow*). (*D*) Once the ureter is laser ablated in front of the trigone, the procedure is complete. Notice the contralateral normal position of the left UVJ (*white arrow*) and the ureteral catheter still within the ureter of the right UVJ after laser ablation is complete.

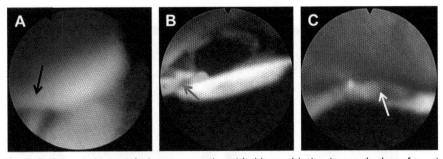

Fig. 9. Endoscopic images during cystoscopic-guided laser ablation in a male dog of a unilateral intramural ectopic ureter. Patient is in dorsal recumbency and a fiber-optic flexible ureteroscope is being used. (*A*) Guide wire (*black arrow*) advanced into the ectopic ureteral opening. (*B*) Laser (*red arrow*) being used to cut the ectopic tissue and advance the ureteral opening into the bladder. (*C*) The new ureteral opening (*white arrow*) after laser ablation is complete and the opening is now in front of the bladder trigone.

URINARY BLADDER AND URETHRA
Perineal Access for Urethrocystoscopy in Male Dogs

Perineal access for urethrocystoscopy is a useful procedure in male dogs heavier than 8 kg and allows for the use of a rigid cystoscopy to gain access into the proximal intrapelvic urethra and bladder, dramatically improving visualization compared with flexible male cystourethroscopy. It also makes interventions like ureteral stenting, CLA-EU, or sclerotherapy/ureteroscopy easier and more effective (**Fig. 10**).

The perineal approach is performed with the patient placed in dorsal recumbency. After flexible urethroscopy to assess the penile and ischial urethra, an 8-Fr Foley catheter is placed into the urethra, with the balloon at the level of the ischium. The urinary bladder is filled with diluted iohexol (50%) and the c-arm fluoroscopy unit is positioned transversely across the dog to project a lateral image. An 18-gauge trocar needle is

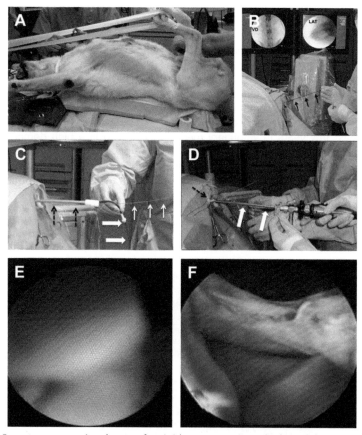

Fig. 10. Percutaneous perineal access for rigid cystoscopy in male dogs. (*A*) Dog in dorsal recumbency with legs taped up and perineal region off the end of the table in a trough. (*B*) 18-gauge needle access (*black arrows*) into the perineal urethra. Notice the fluoroscopy is turned to get a lateral projection while the dog is positioned ventrodorsally. (*C*) Guide wire (*white arrows*) and sheath access (*dashed black arrows*) into the urethra. Urine is being drained out of the sheath (*large white arrows*). (*D*) Rigid cystoscope (*white arrows*) through the sheath (*dashed black arrow*). (*E*) Fiber-optic flexible cystoscope view of a male ectopic ureter with a guide wire in the ureteral orifice. (*F*) Same dog, visualizing the ureteral opening after laser ablation with the rigid cystoscope showing the improved image quality.

placed, under fluoroscopic and ultrasonographic guidance, into the urethra and the needle is aimed to penetrate the balloon of the Foley catheter. A guide wire is advanced into the bladder and using various dilators a tract is made to accept a 14-Fr or 16-Fr peel-away sheath, which accommodates a 2.7-mm rigid cystoscope and allow for various interventions as mentioned earlier. On completion of the intervention, the sheath is removed. The puncture heals by second intension, and the patients are discharged the same day.

In a report of 10 dogs,[12] access time typically took less than 30 minutes, half the cases went home the same day of the procedure, and the only complication encountered was 1 dog leaking urine through the perineal incision 6 hours postoperatively, which did not recur. No long-term complications were identified in any of the dogs with a median follow-up time of ~7 months and in some cases more than 3 years.

Bladder Stone Removal

Bladder stones can be easily removed using various endoscopic techniques.

Studies evaluating traditional surgical removal of stones via cystotomy have shown that 10% to 20% of cases have incomplete surgical removal of stones, and this is likely caused by poor visualization, hemorrhage, or inappropriate technique.[45] Recently, complications associated with traditional surgical cystotomy were reported in 37% to 50% of cases.[45] In addition, there is suggestion of a 40% to 60% rate of stone recurrence, especially when dealing with calcium oxalate, urate, and cystine stones. Various minimally invasive stone retrieval techniques have become more popular over the past few years in veterinary medicine, resulting in a high demand by the veterinary clientele. These options include voiding urohydropropulsion, cystoscopic-guided stone basket retrieval, cystourethroscopic-guided laser lithotripsy, and percutaneous cystolithotomy (PCCL). This article focuses on the endoscopic options.

Cystoscopic-guided stone basket retrieval

Cystoscopic-guided stone basket retrieval (**Fig. 11**) of bladder stones is performed routinely in both male and female dogs and female cats. This procedure is

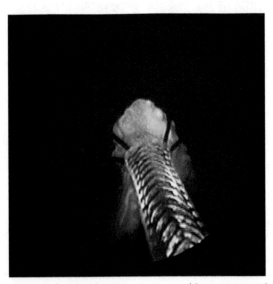

Fig. 11. Endoscopic image of a bladder stone entrapped in a stone retrieval basket.

accomplished by transurethral cystourethroscopy and requires stringent size limitations of both the stone and the patient's urethra. Stones less than 4 mm in female dogs, 2 to 3 mm in most male dogs, and 2 mm in female cats can be routinely retrieved, in the author's experience. This procedure is typically performed on an outpatient basis.

Laser lithotripsy

Laser lithotripsy is a minimally invasive technique that fragments uroliths using cystoscopic guidance intracorporeally using a holmium: YAG laser until the stone fragments are small enough to be voided or basketed through the urethral lumen (**Fig. 12**). The holmium: YAG laser is a pulsed laser that emits light at an infrared wavelength of 2100 nm.[47] The energy is absorbed in less than 0.5 mm of fluid, making it safe to fragment uroliths within the urethra or urinary bladder. For stone fragmentation, laser energy is focused on the urolith surface, directed via cystoscopy, and this results in a photothermal effect, which causes urolith fragmentation. With proper case selection, uroliths can be fragmented and removed in approximately 85% of male dogs and nearly all female dogs.[17]

In the author's experience, animals with larger stone burdens are better suited for a PCCL procedure (see later discussion). Laser lithotripsy should be reserved for female dogs with a few stones or male dogs with only urethral stones.

Percutaneous cystolithotomy

PCCL is a new minimally invasive technique that combines cystic and urethral stone retrieval using cystoscopic and urethroscopic guidance in any size patient, sex, or species and is easy, fast, and effective[48] (**Fig. 13**). This is a particularly useful endoscopic technique to assist in cystourethroscopy when retrograde access is not possible, as in small male dogs and male cats, for urethral stent placement in male cats, for evaluation of the UVJ for upper tract hematuria/IRH, for ureteral stenting in small male dogs, and to retrieve embedded urethral stones in the urethra of small male dogs and male or female cats.

This procedure is performed using a small 1- to 2-cm surgical incision to access the apex of the bladder. A 6-mm screw trocar is then used to cannulate the bladder apex, maintaining a seal to allow for both rigid and flexible antegrade cystoscopy. Saline irrigation is used to maintain bladder distension and visibility. A stone retrieval basket is advanced through the working channel of the cystoscope and guided to remove the larger uroliths, and small fragments are flushed out through the trocar. A flexible cystoscope is then used to visualize the remainder of the urethra, in an antegrade manner.

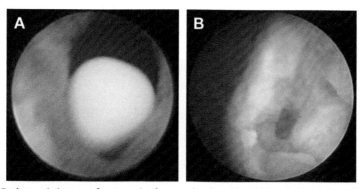

Fig. 12. Endoscopic image of a stone in the proximal urethra (A) and during laser lithotripsy (B) as it is fragmented.

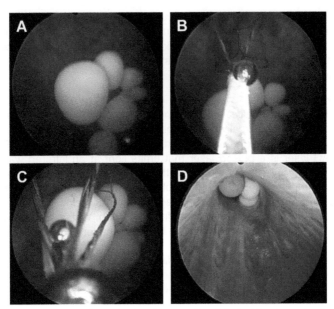

Fig. 13. Cystoscopic images of a male dog during PCCL. (*A*) Bladder stones in the dependent portion of the bladder. (*B*) Stone basket used to remove the stones. (*C*) Basket entrapping the stones. (*D*) Antegrade urethroscopy visualizing the prostatic urethra with a red rubber catheter next to a pile of urethral stones, which can be removed with a stone basket if needed.

These patients are typically discharged the same day as their procedure, once adequate micturition is appreciated.

PCCL is considered the most common minimally invasive bladder stone retrieval method in the author's practice; only 1 of 27 patients had a small fragment left behind on postoperative radiographs, showing improved surgical screening compared with traditional cystotomy.[48]

Endoscopic Polypectomy for Benign Bladder Masses

Endoscopic polypectomy for benign bladder masses can be performed using an endoscopic polypectomy device that can be connected to an electrocautery unit (**Fig. 14**). Urinary bladder polypoid masses can be caused by a benign or malignant process, both of which can cause hematuria, chronic urinary tract infections, dysuria, and potentially, trigonal outflow obstructions. Removal of a polypoid mass can be

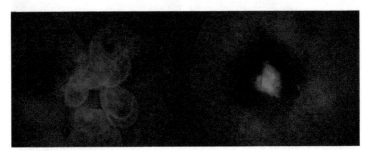

Fig. 14. Large bladder polyp at the apex of the bladder before and after polypectomy.

useful for histopathologic analysis and may have curative results. Masses in the bladder can either be inflammatory polyps, carcinoma in situ, polypoid noninvasive carcinoma, pedunculated invasive carcinoma, or other pedunculated types of masses. Inflammatory polyps are nearly always associated with chronic stone disease or chronic urinary tract infections. Transitional cell carcinoma (TCC) is considered likely if no infection or stone is documented. Invasive TCC, which characterizes more than 90% of veterinary TCC, involving the muscular and often serosal layers, is not considered ideal for local ablative techniques in humans.

If there is a benign polyp, then, the urinary tract infection is treated or the stones are removed. The polyp should resolve on its own over approximately 4 to 6 weeks (depending on the size). If the polyp does not get smaller, or is growing at any point, then, biopsy and polypectomy can be considered.

Polypectomy is accomplished using a snare that is guided through the working channel of the cystoscope, the base of the mass is engaged with the snare, and the electrocautery unit is connected to the snare adaptor. Cautery is applied for ablation of the base. D5W (5% dextrose in water) rather than saline should be used, because it allows for better conduction.

Once all the masses are ablated, a stone retrieval basket is used to remove them from the bladder floor. They should all be submitted for histopathologic evaluation.

Bulking Agent Injections for the Treatment of Urethral Sphincter Mechanism Incompetence

Bulking agent injections for the treatment of urethral sphincter mechanism incompetence (USMI) have been used in women for more than 80 years for the treatment of stress incontinence, and over the past 20 years, this technique has been adapted for use in veterinary medicine. This procedure is typically reserved for dogs that have failed medical management for USMI or are intolerant of side effects associated with the drugs. The principle for using bulking agents is to increase the thickness of the urethral wall in a way that allows coaptation of the urethral mucosa and narrowing of the lumen, creating increased resistance to urine outflow. It also increases the stretch in the urethral muscle fibers, which may allow the muscle to close more effectively. The success of this procedure is often user dependent, so appropriate training is needed.

Various agents have been used like bovine cross-linked collagen (Contigen, Bard Medical, Covington, GA, USA), polytetrafluoroethylene paste (PTFE-Teflon), calcium hydroxylapetite (Coaptite, Boston Scientific, Marlboro, MA, USA), polydimethylsiloxane (PDMS-Macroplastique, Uroplasty, Minnetonka, MN, USA), autologous fat, and carbon-coated zirconium beads (Durasphere, Coloplast, Minneapolis, MN, USA). At this time only calcium hydroxylapetite (Coaptite), carbon-coated beads (Durasphere),

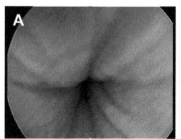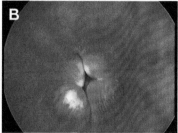

Fig. 15. Bulking agent injections in a female dog with urethral sphincter mechanism incompetence. (*A*) Normal urethra before injection. (*B*) Urethral after injections showing the coaptation of the urethral walls.

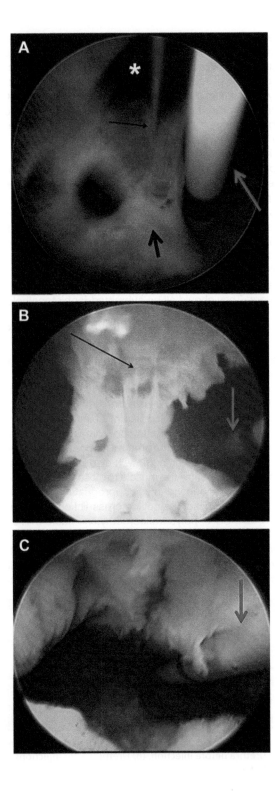

and a newly available cross-linked bovine collagen material (ReGain, Avalon Medical, Minneapolis, MN, USA) are commercially available in the United States.

Glutaraldehyde Cross-Linked Bovine Collagen (Contigen)

Glutaraldehyde cross-linked bovine collagen (Contigen) was the most commonly used bulking agent in dogs and humans, but was recently taken off the market for the treatment of USMI. After injection, this material is vascularized and invaded by fibroblasts, allowing endogenous collagen to be incorporated into the implant, improving implant stabilization. This material is associated with a low complication rate and is relatively easy to inject in a minimally invasive manner, using cystoscopic guidance. In 2005, a study involving 40 dogs reported a 68% continence rate over a mean of 17 months.[49] With the addition of phenylpropanolamine, the continence rate improved to nearly 85%. Complications in this study were minimal and occurred in 15% of dogs, including hematuria, stranguria, and vaginitis, all of which were self-limiting. There are few data on the outcomes after repeated injections, once incontinence returns, but most operators agree that improved responses are common and resumption of continence can be achieved. A newer product, with which clinical trials are under way, called ReGain, is another bovine-derived collagen bulking agent, which may have longer durability in vivo and provide results similar to, or possibly better than, the Contigen product, but the evidence is not yet available.

Regardless of the material, each injection is performed using cystoscopic guidance (**Fig. 15**). Routine cystoscopy is performed to rule out other anatomic anomalies. Once the ureteral openings are identified in their normal anatomic position, the operator identifies the proper location for injection of the bulking agent. This location is typically approximately 2 to 3 cm caudal to the trigone, at a point at which the normal urethral lumen has maximal coaptation and is narrowest. Where the mucosal edges start to meet is a good location for the material to be injected. It is typically recommended to make 3 or 4 blebs at the 2, 6, and 10 o'clock position (or 12, 3, 6, or 9 o'clock). The goal is to have all of the blebs coaptate in the lumen of the urethra so that it appears almost closed but can be expressed.

The main complication with bulking agent injections is temporary urethral outflow tract obstruction, which is rare and short lived. This complication resolves with short-term urethral catheterization if absolutely needed. One should never inject collagen in the face of an active urinary tract infection, so a negative urine culture should always be obtained before this procedure. The author typically treats the patient with 3 days of antibiotics after the procedure, and analgesia is administered on an as-needed basis, similar to that used for routine cystoscopy. Patients can be discharged the same day as the procedure.

Endoscopic Laser Ablation for Vaginal Remnants

Endoscopic laser ablation for vaginal remnants is used for removal of vertical bands at the opening of the vagina, which could be responsible for vaginal pooling, recurrent

Fig. 16. Endoscopic images of a female dog with a persistent paramesonephric remnant (PPMR) before and after laser ablation. Patient is in dorsal recumbency. (*A*) Laser fiber (*black thin arrow*) in contact with the PPMR (*thick black arrow*). A catheter (*red arrow*) is down 1 compartment of the PPMR. The urethral opening (*yellow asterisk*) is visualized above the vagina. (*B*) Laser ablation of the PPMR showing laser fiber (*black thin arrow*) and the urethral catheter (*red arrow*). (*C*) After ablation of the remnant, the vagina is seen to be fully open with the catheter (*red arrow*) visualized.

urinary tract infections, and vaginitis. This condition is most common in dogs with concurrent ectopic ureters, but some dogs have this band of tissue without other anomalies, and treatment has been found to improve clinical signs. A recent study showed that endoscopic laser ablation for vaginal remnants is an effective procedure in maintaining a normal vaginal opening and may improve the risk of recurrent urinary tract infections, vaginitis, and vaginal pooling[16] (**Fig. 16**).

Botulinum-A Toxin Injection for Refractory Detrusor Reflex Dyssynergia or Overactive Bladder

Idiopathic detrusor-urethral dyssynergia (DUD) is a rare condition typically seen in middle-aged large-breed male dogs. It is typically a diagnosis by exclusion. In 1 retrospective study,[50] the prognosis was considered grave, because only 1 of 22 dogs was managed medically and the others were killed. A more recent study described using self-expanding metallic urethral stents in dogs with DUD, with moderate success in a few dogs.

Overactive bladder (OAB), also a rare condition in dogs, is more common in young, large-breed dogs and is typically associated with behavioral issues. This condition can be medically managed with medications like oxybutynin but when refractory can be frustrating.

In human medicine, DUD is also considered rare, but OAB is common. Recent studies have reported success in the use of botulinum-A toxin as a therapy for various voiding disorders, like DUD and OAB. Botulinum toxin is produced by *Clostridium botulinum* and is a neurotoxin that is a presynaptic neuromuscular blocking agent, which results in muscle weakness for up to several months when injected intramuscularly. In the human literature, external urethral sphincter pressure, voiding pressure, and postvoid residual volume were decreased after injection into the external urethral sphincter, lasting 2 to 9 months. For OAB, injections of botulinum-A toxin into the detrusor muscle for detrusor relaxation have been associated with excellent results, improving incontinence. This procedure has been used for DUD in the author's practice; botulinum-A toxin was injected intramuscularly into the urethra using an injection needle via cystoscopic guidance. This procedure was successful for approximately 8 weeks, until the effect subsided.

SUMMARY/DISCUSSION

Endoscopic options for the treatment of various urinary tract diseases has expanded over the past decade in veterinary medicine and is continuing to do so. In this article, only a few of the most common endoscopic procedures performed in veterinary medicine are discussed; these procedures have become more popular in both academic and private practice settings in the last few years. This finding follows a similar trend in human medicine and will likely continue to expand.

It is recommended that operators receive proper training before performing most of the procedures described, because the learning curve is steep and complications should be avoided whenever possible. Training laboratories are available to further develop endourologic skills.

REFERENCES

1. Berent A. New techniques on the horizon: interventional radiology and interventional endoscopy of the urinary tract ('endourology'). J Feline Med Surg 2014; 16(1):51–65.

2. Berent A. Ureteral obstructions in dogs and cats: a review of traditional and new interventional diagnostic and therapeutic options. J Vet Emerg Crit Care (San Antonio) 2011;21(2):86–103.

3. Adams LG, Goldman CK. Extracorporeal shock wave lithotripsy. In: Polzin DJ, Bartges JB, editors. Nephrology and urology of small animals. Ames (IA): Blackwell; 2011. p. 340–8.

4. Adams LG. Nephroliths and ureteroliths: a new stone age. N Z Vet J 2013;61:1–5.

5. Block G, Adams LG, Widmer WR, et al. Use of extracorporeal shock wave lithotripsy for treatment of nephrolithiasis and ureterolithiasis in five dogs. J Am Vet Med Assoc 1996;208:531–6.

6. Donner GS, Ellison GW, Ackerman N, et al. Percutaneous nephrolithotomy in the dog: an experimental study. Vet Surg 1987;16:411–7.

7. Berent A, Weisse C, Bagley D, et al. Endoscopic nephrolithotomy for the treatment of complicated nephrolithiasis in dogs and cats [Abstract]. San Antonio (TX): ACVS; 2013.

8. Berent A, Weisse C, Bagley D, et al. Renal sparing treatment for idiopathic renal hematuria (IRH): endoscopic-guided sclerotherapy. J Am Vet Med Assoc 2013; 242(11):1556–63.

9. Lam N, Berent A, Weisse C, et al. Ureteral stenting for congenital ureteral strictures in a dog. J Am Vet Med Assoc 2012;240(8):983–90.

10. Kuntz J, Berent A, Weisse C, et al. Double pigtail ureteral stenting and renal pelvic lavage for renal-sparing treatment of pyonephrosis in dogs: 13 cases (2008-2012). J Am Vet Med Assoc 2015;246(2):216–25.

11. Pavia P, Berent A, Weisse C, et al. Canine ureteral stenting for benign ureteral obstruction in dogs [Abstract]. San Diego (CA): ACVS; 2014.

12. Weisse C, Berent A. Percutaneous fluoroscopically-assisted perineal approach for rigid cystoscopy in 9 male dogs. Barcelona (Spain): ECVS; 2012.

13. Berent A, Weisse C, Mayhew P, et al. Evaluation of cystoscopic-guided laser ablation of intramural ectopic ureters in 30 female dogs. J Am Vet Med Assoc 2012;240:716–25.

14. Smith AL, Radlinsky MG, Rawlings CA. Cystoscopic diagnosis and treatment of ectopic ureters in female dogs: 16 cases (2005-2008). J Vet Med Assoc 2010; 237(2):191–5.

15. Berent AC, Mayhew PD, Porat-Mosenco Y. Use of cystoscopic-guided laser ablation for treatment of intramural ureteral ectopia in male dogs: four cases (2006-2007). J Am Vet Med Assoc 2008;232(7):1026–34.

16. Burdick S, Berent A, Weisse C, et al. Endoscopic-guided laser ablation of vestibulovaginal defects in 36 dogs. J Am Vet Med Assoc 2014;244(8):944–9.

17. Adams LG, Berent AC, Moore GE, et al. Use of laser lithotripsy for fragmentation of uroliths in dogs: 73 cases (2005-2006). J Am Vet Med Assoc 2008; 232:1680–7.

18. Gookin JL, Stone EA, Spaulding KA, et al. Unilateral nephrectomy in dogs with renal disease: 30 cases (1985-1994). J Am Vet Med Assoc 1996;208:2020–6.

19. King M, Waldron D, Barber D, et al. Effect of nephrotomy on renal function and morphology in normal cats. Vet Surg 2006;35(8):749–58.

20. Adams LG, Williams JC Jr, McAteer JA, et al. In vitro evaluation of canine and feline urolith fragility by shock wave lithotripsy. Am J Vet Res 2005;66:1651–4.

21. Horowitz C, Berent A, Weisse C, et al. Predictors of outcome for cats with ureteral obstructions after interventional management using ureteral stents or a subcutaneous ureteral bypass device. J Feline Med Surg 2013;15(12): 1052–62.

22. Chen KK, Chen MT, Yeh SH, et al. Radionuclide renal function study in various surgical treatments of upper urinary stones. Zhonghua Yi Xue Za Zhi (Taipei) 1992;49(5):319–27.

23. Reis LO, Zani EL, Ikari O, et al. Extracorporeal lithotripsy in children–the efficacy and long-term evaluation of renal parenchyma damage by DMSA-99mTc scintigraphy. Actas Urol Esp 2010;34(1):78–81 [in Spanish].

24. Hubert KC, Palmar JS. Passive dilation by ureteral stenting before ureteroscopy: eliminating the need for active dilation. J Urol 2005;174(3):1079–80.

25. Meretyk S, Gofrit ON, Gafni O, et al. Complete staghorn calculi: random prospective comparison between extracorporeal shock wave lithotripsy monotherapy and combined with percutaneous nephrostolithotomy. J Urol 1997;157:780–6.

26. Al-Hunayan A, Khalil M, Hassabo M, et al. Management of solitary renal pelvic stone: laparoscopic retroperitoneal pyelolithotomy versus percutaneous nephrolithotomy. J Endourol 2011;25(6):975–8.

27. Tawfiek ER, Bagley DH. Ureteroscopic evaluation and treatment of chronic unilateral hematuria. J Urol 1998;160:700–2.

28. Bagley DH, Allen J. Flexible ureteropyeloscopy in the diagnosis of benign essential hematuria. J Urol 1990;143:549–53.

29. Kyles A, Hardie E, Wooden E, et al. Management and outcome of cats with ureteral calculi: 153 cases (1984–2002). J Am Vet Med Assoc 2005;226(6):937–44.

30. Roberts S, Aronson L, Brown D. Postoperative mortality in cats after ureterolithotomy. Vet Surg 2011;40:438–43.

31. Snyder DM, Steffey MA, Mehler SJ, et al. Diagnosis and surgical management of ureteral calculi in dogs: 16 cases (1990-2003). N Z Vet J 2004;53(1):19–25.

32. Kerr WS. Effect of complete ureteral obstruction for one week on kidney function. J Appl Physiol 1954;6:762.

33. Vaughan DE, Sweet RE, Gillenwater JY. Unilateral ureteral occlusion: pattern of nephron repair and compensatory response. J Urol 1973;109:979.

34. Berent A, Weisse C, Bagley D. Ureteral stenting for benign feline ureteral obstructions: technical and clinical outcomes in 79 ureters (2006-2010). J Am Vet Med Assoc 2014;244:559–76.

35. Berent A, Weisse C, Bagley D, et al. The use of a subcutaneous ureteral bypass device for the treatment of feline ureteral obstructions. Seville (Spain): ECVIM; 2011.

36. Steinhaus J, Berent A, Weisse C, et al. Presence of circumcaval ureters and ureteral obstructions in cats. J Vet Intern Med 2015;29(1):63–70.

37. Zimskind PD. Clinical use of long-term indwelling silicone rubber ureteral splints inserted cystoscopically. J Urol 1967;97:840.

38. Uthappa MC. Retrograde or antegrade double-pigtail stent placement for malignant ureteric obstruction? Clin Radiol 2005;60:608.

39. Goldin AR. Percutaneous ureteral splinting. Urology 1977;10(2):165.

40. Lennon GM. Double pigtail ureteric stent versus percutaneous nephrostomy: effects on stone transit and ureteric motility. Eur Urol 1997;31(1):24.

41. Mustafa M. The role of stenting in relieving loin pain following ureteroscopic stone therapy for persisting renal colic with hydronephrosis. Int Urol Nephrol 2007;39(1):91.

42. Yossepowitch O. Predicting the success of retrograde stenting for managing ureteral obstruction. J Urol 2001;166:1746.

43. Nicoli S, Morello E, Martano M, et al. Double-J ureteral stenting in nine cats with ureteral obstruction. Vet J 2012;194(1):60–5.

44. Lane IF, Lappin MR, Seim HB III. Evaluation of results of preoperative urodynamic measurements in 9 dogs with ectopic ureters. J Am Vet Med Assoc 1995;206: 1348–57.
45. Grant DC, Harper TA, Werre SR. Frequency of incomplete urolith removal, complications, and diagnostic imaging following cystotomy for removal of uroliths from the lower urinary tract in dogs: 128 cases (1994-2006). J Am Vet Med Assoc 2010;236(7):763–6.
46. Currao RL, Berent A, Weisse C, et al. Use of a percutaneously controlled urethral hydraulic occluder for treatment of refractory urinary incontinence in 18 female dogs. Vet Surg 2013;42(4):440–7.
47. Wollin TA, Denstedt JD. The holmium laser in urology. J Clin Laser Med Surg 1998;16(1):13.
48. Runge JJ, Berent AC, Mayhew PD. Transvesicular percutaneous cysotolithotomy for the retrieval of cystic and urethral calculi in dogs and cats: 27 cases (2006-2008). J Am Vet Med Assoc 2011;239:344–9.
49. Barth A, Reichler IM, Hubler M, et al. Evaluation of long-term effects of endoscopic injection of collagen into the urethral submucosa for treatment of urethral sphincter incompetence in female dogs: 40 cases (1993-2000). J Am Vet Med Assoc 2005;226:73–6.
50. Diaz Espineira MM, Viehoff FW, Nickel RF. Idiopathic detrusor-urethral dyssynergia in dogs: a retrospective analysis of 22 cases. J Small Anim Pract 1998;39: 264–70.

Complications and Conversion from Endoscopic to Open Surgery

MaryAnn G. Radlinsky, DVM, MS

KEYWORDS

- Endoscopy • Surgery • Complications • Conversion • Minimally invasive

KEY POINTS

- Endoscopic surgery is still a rapidly expanding modality of diagnosis and treatment of small animal patients.
- Hemorrhage, difficulty with visualization, and adjacent tissue trauma seem to be common in the veterinary literature.
- The development of skills, equipment, and minimally invasive means of correcting complications may be of great importance in decreasing the incidence of conversion from endoscopic to open surgery.

COMPLICATIONS

Complications of any endoscopic surgery include complications associated with the purpose of the procedure(s) done. Thus, the clinician MUST be familiar with and capable of performing the procedure via laparotomy, thoracotomy, or sternotomy. Endoscopy is not a substitute for open surgery; attempting an endoscopic procedure that one has not performed via traditional open surgery may not be wise. Conversion to an open approach is the standard rescue for inability to advance or address problems with endoscopy. A full skill set and knowledge of the open approach and procedure must be immediately available in the operative suite, as should be the equipment necessary for open surgery. Conversely, conversion to an open approach is not a failure. Clinicians also should be completely capable of and have the facilities required for aftercare following the procedure, regardless if it is done endoscopically or by a traditional, open approach. The use of endoscopy does not eliminate the need for monitoring and aftercare associated with the procedure, even if the approach is minimally invasive. Expanding one's endoscopic skills to advanced procedures such as pericardectomy, lung lobectomy, mass removal, and so forth should not be attempted

The author has nothing to disclose.
Department of Small Animal Medicine & Surgery, College of Veterinary Medicine, The University of Georgia, 2200 College Station Road, Athens, GA 30602, USA
E-mail address: makorad@gmail.com

Vet Clin Small Anim 46 (2016) 137–145
http://dx.doi.org/10.1016/j.cvsm.2015.07.004
0195-5616/16/$ – see front matter © 2016 Elsevier Inc. All rights reserved.

if 24-hour care is not available to monitor a thoracostomy tube after surgery, which is not unique to endoscopic surgery, nor is its need eliminated by doing the procedure endoscopically.

Anesthetic complications of laparoscopy and thoracoscopy have been discussed elsewhere in this issue. Vigilant monitoring and communication between the surgeon and anesthetist are vital to successful endoscopic endeavors. Establishing a cohesive working team should help to limit and overcome common issues specific to laparoscopy and thoracoscopy related to anesthesia. Hypercarbia and hypoxia may be related to establishment of pneumoperitoneum, pneumothorax, or one-lung ventilation (OLV).[1,2] High intra-abdominal pressure (IAP) of 12 to 15 mm Hg should be required only for trochar-cannula insertion; once all ports are in place, reduce the IAP to 6 to 8 mm Hg to decrease the untoward effects of pneumoperitoneum. Occasionally, insufflation of the thorax is done to increase working space in small patients, particularly in cats.[3] Limit the duration and amount of insufflation to as short a duration as possible and do not exceed 2 mm Hg to decrease the risk of complication associated with insufflation. Establish OLV in the operative suite to avoid inadvertent loss of OLV, to allow thoracoscopic visual confirmation of OLV, and to minimize the duration of OLV and its side effects.[4]

Complications can be associated with port placement and may be limited by visualization of the placement with optical ports or endoscopic placement (Endo Tip port [Karl Storz Endoscopy, Goleta, CA, USA]). Many techniques have been advocated to limit damage to internal structures during port placement. Laparoscopic ports can be placed on establishing pneumoperitoneum with a Veress needle; however, many early reports of laparoscopic techniques were associated with the use of a Veress needle. Hemorrhage, splenic laceration, or hollow organ rupture may occur.[5] A recent report described intercostal Veress needle placement for insufflation, which did not result in organ trauma and may be a nice alternative to traditional Veress needle use.[6] Briefly, with the dog in dorsal recumbency, the Veress needle was placed in the middle or ventral third of the last palpable intercostal space. One or 2 attempts resulted in successful needle placement in 88% of the dogs. Minor complications (subcutaneous emphysema, omental or falciform injury) occurred in 41%. Hepatic or splenic trauma or pneumothorax occurred in 14%. The Hasson technique has been advocated to diminish the risk associated with port placement, and an alteration has been described in which the incision in the linea alba is made only large enough for a large red rubber catheter to be inserted for insufflation, after which a trochar cannula can be inserted. Newer "optical" ports and self-dilating ports also have been advocated for minimization of complications associated with port placement. Threaded ports have become more popular because they allow multiple instrument changes without port dislodgement. One such port (ENDOTIP) can be placed through a small abdominal approach with traction sutures on the body wall similar to the Hasson technique. A very small stab incision through the body wall allows the port to be threaded into the abdomen with a 0° endoscope in its lumen. Visual confirmation of abdominal entry sans trauma can be done, and the port will not be excessively deep in the abdomen due to visualization.

Hemorrhage is possible with any surgical procedure, and endoscopy adds the risk of trauma during instrument passage and motion; the latter may be more dramatic than expected early in the learning curve.[7,8] Instruments should always be passed under visual guidance with a wide field of view until the target is reached, then a smaller, more magnified field can be used. Hemorrhage from intercostal vessels is possible, and may occur on port removal due to loss of compression of the vasculature between the port and rib. Placing ports in an open fashion with blunt obturators may help to decrease the risk of intercostal hemorrhage, which can be severe. Newer devices and surgeon skill allow intraoperative hemorrhage to be managed endoscopically. Direct pressure can be applied with a palpation probe, fan retractor, or dissection tool, limiting small vessel blood loss. Pre-tied loops come in different gauges and suture types and can be placed on structures requiring ligation. Endoscopic clip appliers can be used, as in open surgery, and are available in 5-mm or 10-mm sizes. Numerous vessel-sealing devices are available for controlling hemorrhage in 5-mm to 7-mm vessels. Care should be taken to avoid collateral trauma to adjacent structures. Be aware that the divider included in sealer-dividers transects all tissue in the jaws of the instrument, and tissue at the junction of the jaws of the device has not been sealed. Transection of this unsealed tissue can result in hemorrhage. Care also should be taken to avoid contact of sealing devices with adjacent tissues, which can result in thermal damage.

The requirement of pneumoperitoneum for laparoscopy can result in accumulation of CO_2 in undesired tissues, including the subcutis, body wall, omental bursa, and pleural space (in the case of undiagnosed diaphragmatic hernia). Monitor for subcutaneous emphysema to ensure that it does not become significant and cause patient discomfort on recovery from general anesthesia. Accumulation of gas in the body wall or omental bursa can cause difficulties with access or visualization, leading to conversion to open surgery.

Late complications are similar to those associated with the approach for open surgery, and include herniation through the port sites, infection, dehiscence, seroma, bruising, and, particular to endoscopy, port site metastasis.[9] The manipulation of tumors alone can result in port site metastasis, the etiology of which remains unknown. Because port site can become affected by tumor and potentially infected, it is recommended to place all tissues removed from the abdomen or chest in specimen-retrieval bags to minimize contact with the port site.

Pneumoperitoneum and pneumothorax should be eliminated at the end of laparoscopy and thoracoscopy, respectively. Care should be taken to avoid inadvertent pulmonary trauma during instrument introduction and removal, as well as during manipulation of the target structures. Fan retractors should be used with caution; entrapment of lung between the blades can result in trauma. A thoracostomy tube should be placed as would be done with open surgery to allow removal of air from the chest and to monitor for hemorrhage or reaccumulation of air after surgery.

CONVERSION TO OPEN SURGERY

Conversion to an open approach is not a failure of the endoscopic procedure and may be done on an elective or emergent basis. Elective conversions are done without the presence of a complication and may be due to concerns about the duration of the procedure, safety for the patient, poor visualization (often due to the presence of fat, adhesions, or abnormal anatomy), lesions too large for endoscopic removal, or failure to progress, which may relate to patient factors leading to poor visualization or surgeon experience. Emergent conversions are required when complications cannot be managed endoscopically.

Conversion may be due to patient, equipment, or surgeon factors. Patient-related factors include high body condition score, gender, age, disease, and anatomic factors.[7] Fat, minor hemorrhage, and adhesions may limit the ability to complete a procedure endoscopically, resulting in conversion to open surgery. Other patient-related factors include concurrent diseases, inability to tolerate pneumoperitoneum, or OLV. Equipment issues that cannot be addressed quickly also may result in conversion to open surgery. For laparoscopy, inability to maintain pneumoperitoneum may limit working space and result in conversion. Large mass lesions also may limit visualization within the thorax, even if the lesion is not being removed, as with pericardectomy for heart base tumors. Surgeon experience and training also may lead to conversion.

REVIEW OF LITERATURE

Articles describing veterinary laparoscopic efforts were evaluated for complications and conversion to open surgery. The articles included ovariectomy, adrenalectomy, treatment of hemorrhage, development of techniques, descriptive studies or reviews, embryo transfer, gastropexy, biopsy study, lift laparoscopy, lymph node removal, and nephrectomy.[10–40] Intraoperative complications included blood loss (9 studies), splenic laceration (4), and subcutaneous emphysema (2); and each of the following were reported in only 1 study: adhesions interfering with visualization, leakage of CO_2 around ports, fat impairing visualization, specimen-retrieval bag laceration, difficulty extracting ovaries.[22–24,38]

Specific intraoperative complications not resulting in conversion occurred in 0.09% of 739 animals described in the literature that included intraoperative complications.[10–40] Descriptions of the development of new techniques were not included if the technique was not yet widely used because of the higher than expected rate of complications in development of new techniques in experimental study. The most commonly listed complication was intraoperative hemorrhage (0.02%), splenic trauma (0.01%), and subcutaneous emphysema (0.05%); rarely reported were fat interference with visualization (1 case), trauma to the specimen to be collected (3), problems related to port position (3), trouble retrieving a specimen (2), and equipment-related or anesthesia-related difficulty (1 each). Realizing that all intraoperative difficulties may not have been included, and the exclusion of development of techniques that may have led to complications not associated with clinical use of endoscopy, these intraoperative complications seem typical for those related to endoscopic surgery. Furthermore, retrospective studies may not include intraoperative complications that were readily and rapidly addressed without conversion.

Postoperative complications included inflammation of port sites (2 studies) and vomiting after gastropexy (2), and 1 study each reported decreased appetite, dehiscence at a port site, and port site seroma formation.[21,28,35,36] All of the complications described are not uncommon following any open surgery, and infection is reportedly less with endoscopic surgery compared with open surgery.

Similar evaluation of thoracoscopic surgery in small animals included articles reporting lung lobectomy, thoracic duct ligation, pericardectomy, lymph node removal, cisterna chyli ablation, pyothorax, biopsy techniques, right atrial mass removal, diagnosis of pleural effusion, treatment of persistent right aortic arch, and mass removal.[3,4,41–75] Intraoperative complications included hemorrhage (3 studies), phrenic nerve trauma (2), and problems with OLV (3), and 1 study each reported hypoventilation, prolongation of anesthesia, and postoperative pneumothorax. Problems with OLV included hypoxemia and intolerance (2 studies), and 1 each loss of OLV and inability to establish OLV. Postoperative complications included seroma (reported in 3 studies) and air leakage (2), and 1 study each reported hypoventilation on recovery, recurrence of pneumothorax, pulmonary thromboembolism, lameness, and port site dehiscence.[41,42,50,62,73,74]

Specific intraoperative complications not resulting in conversion to open surgery occurred in 5.2% in studies that included intraoperative complications; again, development of new techniques was not included if the techniques were not widely accepted because a higher than normal complication rate would be encountered in those studies.[3,4,41–46,54–65,69–74] The most commonly reported complication was pulmonary trauma (1%) followed by anesthetic-related issues (0.5%). Leakage of dye also was encountered in the sealing of the thoracic duct in 1 study.

Conversion from laparoscopy to laparotomy also was identified in studies, and ranged from 0% to 21%.[6,10–40] Reasons for conversion included hemorrhage (4 studies), leakage from a hollow viscous (2), and study reported need for resection anastomosis, unidentified reason, complex adhesions, anesthetic reasons, technical error, unexpected mass lesion, overdistension of the gastrointestinal tract interfering with progression, slow progression of the procedure, and too large a mass for removal.[22–24,38]

Conversion from thoracoscopy to lateral thoracotomy or sternotomy was identified in studies and ranged from 0% to 50%, including all studies reporting thoracoscopy.[3,4,9,41–74] This provides the worst-case scenario for all endoscopic procedures of the chest. Reasons for conversion included hemorrhage, reported in 5 studies, inability to identify a lesion (3 studies), limited visualization (3 studies), loss of OLV (2 studies), and 1 study each reported prolonged surgery time, adjacent tissue trauma, and poor access as reasons for conversion to open surgery.[4,43,50,58,65,70,73]

In conclusion, endoscopic surgery is still a rapidly expanding modality of diagnosis and treatment of small animal patients. Hemorrhage, difficulty with visualization, and adjacent tissue trauma seem to be common in the veterinary literature. The development of skills, equipment, and minimally invasive means of correcting complications may be of great importance in decreasing the incidence of conversion from endoscopic to open surgery; however, conversion to an open approach should never be seen as a failure. Conversion should be considered at any time that it is of the greatest benefit for the patient. This concept is important enough to warrant discussion with the owner before surgery and acceptance of the need to convert without further consultation during the procedure.

REFERENCES

1. Kudnig ST, Monnet E, Riquelme M, et al. Effect of positive end-expiratory pressure on oxygen delivery during 1-lung ventilation for thoracoscopy in normal dogs. Vet Surg 2006;35:534–42.
2. Cantwell SL, Duke T, Walsh PJ, et al. One-lung versus two-lung ventilation in the closed-chest anesthetized dog: a comparison of cardiopulmonary parameters. Vet Surg 2000;29:365–73.
3. Mayhew PD, Pascoe PJ, Shilo-Benjamini Y, et al. Effect of one-lung ventilation with or without low-pressure carbon dioxide insufflation on cardiorespiratory variables in cats undergoing thoracoscopy. Vet Surg 2015;44(Suppl 1):15–22.
4. Lansdowne JL, Monnet E, Twedt DC, et al. Thoracoscopic lung lobectomy for treatment of lung tumors in dogs. Vet Surg 2005;34:530–5.
5. Buote NJ, Kovak-McClaran JR, Schold JD. Conversion from diagnostic laparoscopy to laparotomy: risk factors and occurrence. Vet Surg 2011;40:106–14.
6. Fiorbianco V, Skalicky M, Doerner J, et al. Right intercostal insertion of a Veress needle for laparoscopy in dogs. Vet Surg 2012;41:367–73.
7. McClaran JK, Buote NJ. Complications and need for conversion to laparotomy in small animals. Vet Clin North Am Small Anim Pract 2009;39:941–51.
8. Radlinsky MG. Complications and need for conversion from thoracoscopy to thoracotomy in small animals. Vet Clin North Am Small Anim Pract 2009;39:977–84.

9. Brisson BA, Reggeti F, Bienzle D. Portal site metastasis of invasive mesothelioma after diagnostic thoracoscopy in a dog. J Am Vet Med Assoc 2006;229:980–3.

10. Shariati E, Bakhtiari J, Khalaj A, et al. Comparison between two portal laparoscopy and open surgery for ovariectomy in dogs. Vet Res Forum 2014;5:219–23.

11. Smith RR, Mayhew PD, Berent AC. Laparoscopic adrenalectomy for management of a functional adrenal tumor in a cat. J Am Vet Med Assoc 2012;241: 368–72.

12. Naan EC, Kirpensteijn J, Dupre GP, et al. Innovative approach to laparoscopic adrenalectomy for treatment of unilateral adrenal gland tumors in dogs. Vet Surg 2013;42:710–5.

13. Lambo CA, Grahm RA, Lyons LA, et al. Comparative fertility of freshly collected vs frozen-thawed semen with laparoscopic oviductal artificial insemination in domestic cats. Reprod Domest Anim 2012;47(Suppl 6):284–8.

14. Koenraadt A, Stegen L, Bosmans T, et al. Laparoscopic treatment of persistent inguinal haemorrhage after prescrotal orchiectomy in a dog. J Small Anim Pract 2014;55:427–30.

15. Sherwinter DA. A novel retraction instrument improves the safety of single-incision laparoscopic cholecystectomy in an animal model. J Laparoendosc Adv Surg Tech A 2012;22:158–61.

16. Mathon DH, Dossin O, Palierne S, et al. A laparoscopic-sutured gastropexy technique in dogs: mechanical and functional evaluation. Vet Surg 2009;38: 967–74.

17. Secchi P, Filho HC, Scussel Feranti JP, et al. Laparoscopic-assisted incisional colopexy by two portals access in a domestic cat with recurrent rectal prolapse. J Feline Med Surg 2012;14:169–70.

18. Zhang SX, Wang HB, Zhang JT, et al. Laparoscopic colopexy in dogs. J Vet Med Sci 2013;75:1161–6.

19. Runge JJ, Mayhew PD, Case JB, et al. Single-port laparoscopic cryptorchidectomy in dogs and cats: 25 cases (2009-2014). J Am Vet Med Assoc 2014;245: 1258–65.

20. Dupré G, Čoudek K. Laparoscopic-assisted placement of a peritoneal dialysis catheter with partial omentectomy and omentopexy in dogs: an experimental study. Vet Surg 2013;42:579–85.

21. Spah CE, Elkins AD, Wehrenberg A, et al. Evaluation of two novel self-anchoring barbed sutures in a prophylactic laparoscopic gastropexy compared with intracorporeal tied knots. Vet Surg 2013;42:932–42.

22. Fransson BA, Grubb TL, Perez TE, et al. Cardiorespiratory changes and pain response of lift laparoscopy compared to capnoperitoneum laparoscopy in dogs. Vet Surg 2014;44(Suppl 1):7–14.

23. Fransson BA, Ragle CA. Lift laparoscopy in dogs and cats: 12 cases (2008-2009). J Am Vet Med Assoc 2011;239:1574–9.

24. Petre SL, McClaran JK, Bergman PJ, et al. Safety and efficacy of laparoscopic hepatic biopsy in dogs: 80 cases (2004-2009). J Am Vet Med Assoc 2012;240: 181–5.

25. Steffey MA, Daniel L, Mayhew PD, et al. Laparoscopic extirpation of the medial iliac lymph nodes in normal dogs. Vet Surg 2014;44(Suppl 1):59–65.

26. Kim YK, Park SJ, Lee SY, et al. Laparoscopic nephrectomy in dogs: an initial experience of 16 experimental procedures. Vet J 2013;198:513–7.

27. Kim YK, Lee SS, Suh EH, et al. Sprayed intraperitoneal bupivacaine reduces early postoperative pain behavior and biochemical stress response after laparoscopic ovariohysterectomy in dogs. Vet J 2012;191:188–92.

28. Pope JF, Knowles T. The efficacy of n-butyl-cyanoacrylate tissue adhesive for closure of canine laparoscopic ovariectomy port site incisions. J Small Anim Pract 2013;54:190–4.
29. Hartman MJ, Monnet E, Kirberger RM, et al. Laparoscopic sterilization of the African lioness (*Panthera leo*). Vet Surg 2013;42:559–64.
30. Lee JY, Kim MC. Comparison of oxidative stress status in dogs undergoing laparoscopic and open ovariectomy. J Vet Med Sci 2014;76:273–6.
31. Öhlund M, Höglund O, Olsson U, et al. Laparoscopic ovariectomy in dogs: a comparison of the LigaSure™ and the SonoSurg™ systems. J Small Anim Pract 2011;52:290–4.
32. Manassero M, Leperlier D, Vallefuoco R, et al. Laparoscopic ovariectomy in dogs using a single-port multiple-access device. Vet Rec 2012;171:69.
33. Kim YK, Lee SY, Park SJ, et al. Feasibility of single-portal access laparoscopic ovariectomy in 17 cats. Vet Rec 2011;169:179.
34. Runge JJ, Curcillo PG 2nd, King SA, et al. Initial application of reduced port surgery using the single port access technique for laparoscopic canine ovariectomy. Vet Surg 2012;41:803–6.
35. Rivier P, Furneaux R, Viguier E. Combined laparoscopic ovariectomy and laparoscopic-assisted gastropexy in dogs susceptible to gastric dilatation-volvulus. Can Vet J 2011;52:62–6.
36. Adamovich-Rippe KN, Mayhew PD, Runge JJ, et al. Evaluation of laparoscopic-assisted ovariohysterectomy for treatment of canine-36. Vet Surg 2013;42:572–8.
37. Cho YB, Park CH, Kim HC, et al. Single-incision laparoscopic surgery in a survival animal model using a transabdominal magnetic anchoring system. Surg Endosc 2011;25:3934–8.
38. Runge JJ, Mayhew PD. Evaluation of single port access gastropexy and ovariectomy using articulating instruments and angled telescopes in dogs. Vet Surg 2013;42:807–13.
39. Radhakrishnan A, Mayhew PD. Laparoscopic splenic biopsy in dogs and cats: 15 cases (2006-2008). J Am Anim Hosp Assoc 2013;49:41–5.
40. Khalaj A, Bakhtiari J, Niasari-Naslaji A. Comparison between single and three portal laparoscopic splenectomy in dogs. BMC Vet Res 2012;8:161.
41. Levionnois OL, Bergadano A, Schatzmann U. Accidental entrapment of an endobronchial blocker tip by a surgical stapler during selective ventilation for lung lobectomy in a dog. Vet Surg 2006;35:82–5.
42. Brissot HN, Dupre GP, Bouvy BM, et al. Thoracoscopic treatment of bullous emphysema in 3 dogs. Vet Surg 2003;32:524–9.
43. Case JB, Mayhew PD, Singh A. Evaluation of video-assisted thoracic surgery for treatment of spontaneous pneumothorax and pulmonary bullae in dogs. Vet Surg 2015;44(Suppl 1):31–8.
44. Sakals S, Schmiedt CW, Radlinsky MG. Comparison and description of trans-diaphragmatic and abdominal minimally invasive cisterna chyli ablation in dogs. Vet Surg 2011;40:795–801.
45. Haimel G, Liehmann L, Dupré G. Thoracoscopic en bloc thoracic duct sealing and partial pericardectomy for the treatment of chylothorax in two cats. J Feline Med Surg 2012;14:928–31.
46. Mayhew PD, Culp WT, Mayhew KN, et al. Minimally invasive treatment of idiopathic chylothorax in dogs by thoracoscopic thoracic duct ligation and subphrenic pericardiectomy: 6 cases (2007-2010). J Am Vet Med Assoc 2012;241:904–9.
47. Daly CM, Swalec-Tobias K, Tobias AH, et al. Cardiopulmonary effects of intrathoracic insufflation in dogs. J Am Anim Hosp Assoc 2002;38:515–20.

48. Steffey MA, Daniel L, Mayhew PD, et al. Video-assisted thoracoscopic extirpation of the tracheobronchial lymph nodes in dogs. Vet Surg 2015;44(Suppl 1):50–8.

49. Peláez MJ, Jolliffe C. Thoracoscopic foreign body removal and right middle lung lobectomy to treat pyothorax in a dog. J Small Anim Pract 2012;53:240–4.

50. Mayhew PD, Hunt GB, Steffey MA, et al. Evaluation of short-term outcome after lung lobectomy for resection of primary lung tumors via video-assisted thoracoscopic surgery or open thoracotomy in medium- to large-breed dogs. J Am Vet Med Assoc 2013;243:681–8.

51. García F, Prandi D, Peña T, et al. Examination of the thoracic cavity and lung lobectomy by means of thoracoscopy in dogs. Can Vet J 1998;39:285–91.

52. Mayhew PD, Culp WT, Pascoe PJ, et al. Use of the Ligasure vessel-sealing device for thoracoscopic peripheral lung biopsy in healthy dogs. Vet Surg 2012;41: 523–8.

53. Mayhew PD, Culp WT, Pascoe PJ, et al. Evaluation of blind thoracoscopic-assisted placement of three double-lumen endobronchial tube designs for one-lung ventilation in dogs. Vet Surg 2012;41:664–70.

54. Adami C, Axiak S, Rytz U, et al. Alternating one lung ventilation using a double lumen endobronchial tube and providing CPAP to the non-ventilated lung in a dog. Vet Anaesth Analg 2011;38:70–6.

55. Bauquier SH, Culp WT, Lin RC, et al. One-lung ventilation using a wire-guided endobronchial blocker for thoracoscopic pericardial fenestration in a dog. Can Vet J 2010;51:1135–8.

56. Borenstein N, Behr L, Chetboul V, et al. Minimally invasive patent ductus arteriosus occlusion in 5 dogs. Vet Surg 2004;33:309–13.

57. Case JB, Maxwell M, Aman A, et al. Outcome evaluation of a thoracoscopic pericardial window procedure or subtotal pericardectomy via thoracotomy for the treatment of pericardial effusion in dogs. J Am Vet Med Assoc 2013;242: 493–8.

58. Atencia S, Doyle RS, Whitley NT. Thoracoscopic pericardial window for management of pericardial effusion in 15 dogs. J Small Anim Pract 2013;54:564–9.

59. Crumbaker DM, Rooney MB, Case JB. Thoracoscopic subtotal pericardiectomy and right atrial mass resection in a dog. J Am Vet Med Assoc 2010;237:551–4.

60. Bernard F, Kudnig ST, Monnet E. Hemodynamic effects of interpleural lidocaine and bupivacaine combination in anesthetized dogs with and without an open pericardium. Vet Surg 2006;35:252–8.

61. Dupré GP, Corlouer JP, Bouvy B. Thoracoscopic pericardectomy performed without pulmonary exclusion in 9 dogs. Vet Surg 2001;30:21–7.

62. Mayhew KN, Mayhew PD, Sorrell-Raschi L, et al. Thoracoscopic subphrenic pericardectomy using double-lumen endobronchial intubation for alternating one-lung ventilation. Vet Surg 2009;38:961–6.

63. Walsh PJ, Remedios AM, Ferguson JF, et al. Thoracoscopic versus open partial pericardectomy in dogs: comparison of postoperative pain and morbidity. Vet Surg 1999;28:472–9.

64. Jackson J, Richter KP, Launer DP. Thoracoscopic partial pericardiectomy in 13 dogs. J Vet Intern Med 1999;13:529–33.

65. Kovak JR, Ludwig LL, Bergman PJ, et al. Use of thoracoscopy to determine the etiology of pleural effusion in dogs and cats: 18 cases (1998-2001). J Am Vet Med Assoc 2002;221:990–4.

66. Jerram RM, Fossum TW, Berridge BR, et al. The efficacy of mechanical abrasion and talc slurry as methods of pleurodesis in normal dogs. Vet Surg 1999;28: 322–32.

67. Grand JG, Bureau SC. Video-assisted thoracoscopic surgery for pneumothorax induced by migration of a K-wire to the chest. J Am Anim Hosp Assoc 2011; 47:268–75.

68. Plesman R, Johnson M, Rurak S, et al. Thoracoscopic correction of a congenital persistent right aortic arch in a young cat. Can Vet J 2011;52:1123–8.

69. Isakow K, Fowler D, Walsh P. Video-assisted thoracoscopic division of the ligamentum arteriosum in two dogs with persistent right aortic arch. J Am Vet Med Assoc 2000;217:1333–6.

70. MacPhail CM, Monnet E, Twedt DC. Thoracoscopic correction of persistent right aortic arch in a dog. J Am Anim Hosp Assoc 2001;37:577–81.

71. Ployart S, Libermann S, Doran I, et al. Thoracoscopic resection of right auricular masses in dogs: 9 cases (2003-2011). J Am Vet Med Assoc 2013;242:237–41.

72. Allman DA, Radlinsky MG, Ralph AG, et al. Thoracoscopic thoracic duct ligation and thoracoscopic pericardectomy for treatment of chylothorax in dogs. Vet Surg 2010;39:21–7.

73. Radlinsky MG, Mason DE, Biller DS, et al. Thoracoscopic visualization and ligation of the thoracic duct in dogs. Vet Surg 2002;31:138–46.

74. Leasure CS, Ellison GW, Roberts JF, et al. Occlusion of the thoracic duct using ultrasonically activated shears in six dogs. Vet Surg 2011;40:802–10.

75. Mayhew PD, Friedberg JS. Video-assisted thoracoscopic resection of noninvasive thymomas using one-lung ventilation in two dogs. Vet Surg 2008;37:756–62.

Advances in Video-Assisted Thoracic Surgery, Thoracoscopy

Joseph Brad Case, DVM, MS

KEYWORDS

- Thoracoscopy • Video-assisted thoracic surgery • Pericardectomy
- Lung lobectomy • Pleural • One-lung ventilation • Pneumothorax

KEY POINTS

- Patient selection is critical, and general and specific contraindications exist.
- Anesthetic management can be challenging and may require an anesthesiologist if one-lung ventilation (OLV) is to be used.
- Elective and emergent conversion may be necessary, and the operating surgeon must be willing to convert if patient safety or the success of the surgery is in question.
- Perioperative management is similar to cases undergoing planned thoracotomy.

PERICARDIAL EFFUSION AND NEOPLASIA

Pathologic pericardial effusion can result from malignancy, infectious, or idiopathic etiologies. Among malignant causes, hemangiosarcoma of the right auricular appendage is most common, but aortic body chemodectoma and diffuse mesothelioma are also seen. Malignant pericardial effusion is diagnosed in about 70% and idiopathic pericardial effusion is seen in about 20% to 30% of dogs presenting for pathologic pericardial effusion.[1,2] When the volume of effusion becomes significant, a reduction in end diastolic volume and cardiac output results, a condition referred to as cardiac tamponade. One of the most commonly performed video-assisted thoracic surgery (VATS) procedures in dogs is pericardectomy.[2–6] The objective of pericardectomy is to excise enough pericardium to eliminate tamponade and to obtain a histologic diagnosis of the patient's condition (**Table 1**).

The surgeon must decide how much pericardium to excise when considering pericardectomy. In palliative cases, such as those associated with neoplastic effusions, a 4 × 4 cm pericardial window seems to be adequate unless right auriculectomy is being

The author has nothing to disclose.

Small Animal Surgery, College of Veterinary Medicine, University of Florida, 2015 Southwest 16th Avenue, Gainesville, FL 32608, USA

E-mail address: caseb@ufl.edu

Vet Clin Small Anim 46 (2016) 147–169
http://dx.doi.org/10.1016/j.cvsm.2015.07.005
0195-5616/16/$ – see front matter

Table 1
VATS indications and contraindications

Indications	Contraindications
Pericardial effusion and neoplasia	Lack of training and instrumentation
Cranial mediastinal mass resection	Unstable patient
Pulmonary neoplasia	Lack of anesthetic support
Pulmonary blebs and bullae	Large masses or lesions
Chylothorax	—
Vascular ring anomaly	—

considered.[2,3,6,7] With presumed idiopathic cases, a complete pericardioscopic evaluation is necessary to reduce the chance of a missed diagnosis and a larger pericardectomy is indicated.[2,8] Because masses are common on the right auricle and heart base (**Fig. 1**), the surgeon must have adequate experience and understanding of the pericardial anatomy before performing pericardoscopy, auriculectomy, or epicardial biopsy.[6,7]

The combination of a pericardial window and pericardial fillet has recently been described.[9] The pericardial fillet facilitates exposure of most of the intrapericardiac anatomy without the need for subphrenic pericardectomy.[9] Pericardial fillet is performed by creating several individual incisions, from ventral to dorsal toward the phrenic nerves, following excision of an approximate 4 × 4 cm apical window (**Fig. 2**). The orientation of the window (and fillet if performed) is likely not as important as performing a thorough pericardioscopic assessment. This is particularly important in presumed idiopathic cases, because it is possible for small nodules and masses to be identified on endoscopy around the heart base (**Fig. 3**) in dogs with a preoperative negative echocardiogram.[2,8] In this scenario, some dogs are tentatively diagnosed with an idiopathic pericardial effusion. If a representative epicardial (**Fig. 4**) sample is not obtained during pericardioscopy and/or if the pericardial sample obtained is not representative of the underlying disease, then a missed diagnosis and lost opportunity for disease-specific medical therapy occurs.

Right auricular mass resection in combination with pericardectomy has recently been described in nine dogs.[6] One dog died during surgery from hemorrhage but eight

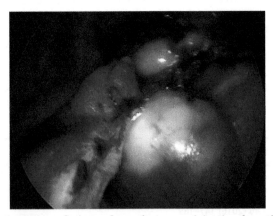

Fig. 1. Intraoperative image of a large chemodectoma originating from the heart base in a dog undergoing VATS pericardectomy.

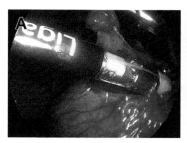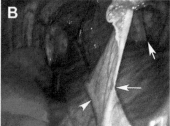

Fig. 2. Intraoperative image of a dog undergoing VATS pericardial window (*A*) and pericardial fillet (*B*). The arrow heads show the phrenic nerve. (*Courtesy of* Mary Ann Radlinsky, DVM, MS, DACVS, University of Georgia, Athens, GA.)

dogs underwent successful resection of the atrial mass. Dogs with masses limited to the tip of the atrial appendage were considered to be good candidates for a VATS auricular resection.[6] The benefits of performing appendage resection in conjunction with pericardectomy are to obtain histologic diagnosis and to reduce the risk of hemorrhage from atrial rupture.[6,7]

CRANIAL MEDIASTINAL NEOPLASIA

Cranial mediastinal neoplasia is uncommon in dogs and cats. However, when observed, the most likely diagnoses are lymphoma, thymoma, and less commonly thymic carcinoma. Other neoplasms of the cranial mediastinum have also been described.[10] Dogs with thymic lymphoma are managed medically, whereas dogs with other neoplasms, such as thymoma, are treated surgically. Traditionally, resection of cranial mediastinal masses (CMMs) has been accomplished via median sternotomy or intercostal thoracotomy.[11–14] Recently, a VATS approach to CMM resection in two dogs was reported.[15] A VATS approach to CMM resection is feasible and associated with low operative morbidity, although ultimate prognosis depends on the underlying disease. For example, dogs with myasthenia gravis and megaesophagus have a poor

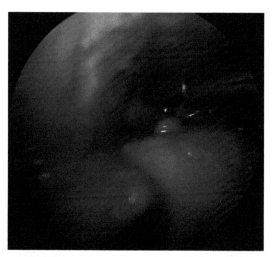

Fig. 3. Multiple small nodules on the aortic root and right auricle in a dog undergoing pericardectomy and epicardial biopsy for presumed idiopathic pericardial effusion. The pericardium histopathology showed pericarditis and the epicardial biopsy revealed mesothelioma.

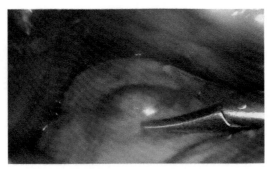

Fig. 4. A dog with presumed idiopathic pericardial effusion undergoing epicardial biopsy at the heart base after pericardectomy.

short-term outcome.[11,14,16] Preoperative computed tomography (**Fig. 5**) is strongly advised in preoperative case selection for confirmation of noninvasiveness. Dogs greater than 20 kg with noninvasive masses and masses with a diameter less than 7 cm or an approximate volume less than 300 cm³ seem to be good candidates for a CMM resection.[16]

Dogs undergoing VATS CMM resection are positioned in dorsal recumbency (**Fig. 6**). Ports are placed as previously described.[15] The fourth intercostal space facilitates finger-assisted retraction and ultimately extraction of the mass following dissection.

Once all ports have been placed and the mediastinum has been dissected, the mass is explored laterally and dorsally to ensure no adhesions or infiltration of major vessels, such as the cranial vena cava, brachycephalic artery, and left subclavian artery (**Fig. 7**). It is common for the internal thoracic vessels (**Fig. 8**) to be adhered and infiltrative to the mass but careful dissection allows separation of these vessels without compromise of the tumor capsule. Dissection of the mass begins ventrally to separate the mass from the internal thoracic vessels. This is usually performed with a combination of sharp and blunt dissection using VATS Kelly and right-angle dissecting forceps in addition to a vessel-sealing device. Perhaps the most critical aspect of the dissection is ventral retraction of the mass away from the phrenic nerves and major cardiac vessels (eg, vena cava and brachycephalic artery) during dissection dorsal to the mass. This is accomplished with sponge forceps, Babcock forceps, fan retractors, and/or transthoracic digital retraction (**Fig. 9**). Once the mass has been dissected free, a sterile specimen retrieval bag is used to remove the mass from the thoracic

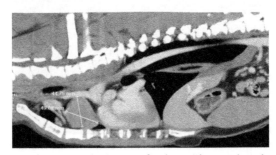

Fig. 5. Sagital computed tomography image of a dog with a noninvasive thymoma. Notice the close association of the mass with the internal thoracic vessels and brachycephalic trunk.

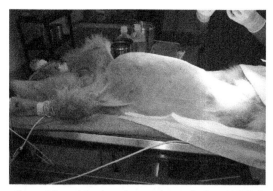

Fig. 6. A dog correctly positioned in dorsal recumbency before VATS thymectomy.

cavity (**Fig. 10**). With the required training and experience with VATS, CMM resection is feasible and associated with low operative morbidity. A recent abstract revealed that only 1 out of 18 dogs undergoing VATS CMM resection did not survive surgery.[16] The complication in this case was laceration of the cranial vena cava during dissection dorsal to the mass.

PERSISTENT RIGHT AORTIC ARCH AND LEFT LIGAMENTUM ARTERIOSUM

Vascular ring anomalies are uncommon malformations of the aortic arches during fetal development, which result in some degree of constriction of the esophagus. The most common vascular ring anomaly seen in dogs is the persistent right aortic arch with a left ligamentum. This malformation causes the esophagus to become constricted between the ligamentum arteriosum, right-sided descending aorta and pulmonary artery, and the trachea. Surgical transection of the ligamentum is

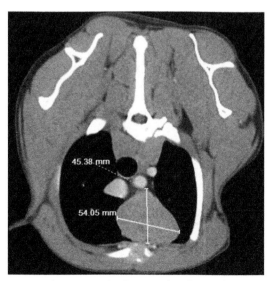

Fig. 7. Transverse computed tomography image of a dog with a noninvasive thymoma. Notice the cranial vena cava, brachycephalic trunk, and subclavian vessels immediately dorsal to the mass.

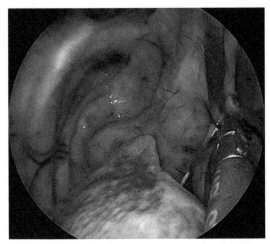

Fig. 8. Intraoperative image of a dog undergoing VATS thymectomy. The right-angle forceps are useful in dissecting the internal thoracic vessels away from the mass.

necessary and the prognosis is good to excellent in most cases, although some degree of esophageal dilation may persist.[17]

Dogs are young and typically malnourished at the time of diagnosis and are therefore not ideal surgical candidates. Effort should be made to encourage nutritional support as best possible before surgical intervention, although treatment should not be delayed for an extended period of time. Because affected dogs usually only tolerate gruel diets, small-volume elevated feedings can be continued up to 12 hours before surgery to reduce the chance of hypoglycemia. A VATS approach to ligamentum transection has been reported in one, two, and 14 dogs.[18–20]

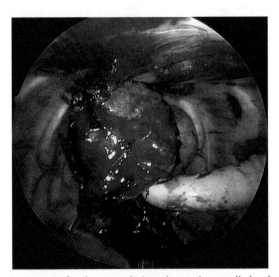

Fig. 9. Intraoperative image of a thymoma being elevated ventrally by the surgeon's finger to aid in dorsal dissection. Ventral elevation is critical during dissection to reduce the risk of injury to a great vessel.

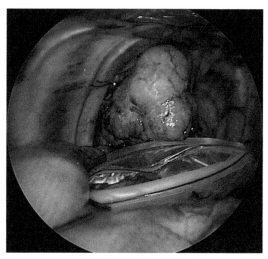

Fig. 10. Intraoperative image of a thymoma being placed in a specimen retrieval bag for removal from the thorax.

The left hemithorax is clipped completely from dorsal to ventral across midline and from the caudal cervical region to the cranial abdomen. Dogs are positioned in right lateral recumbency (**Fig. 11**) with the dorsal spine elevated approximately 15°. Three intercostal ports are used for ligamentum transection. The author's preference is to use two 3.5-mm pediatric threaded cannulas in the dorsal and ventral seventh or eighth intercostal spaces and a 1-mL syringe case in between the two pediatric ports. A 3-mm telescope is inserted through one of the threaded cannulas and a metered blunt probe is placed through the other for exploration and palpation of the ligamentum. A flexible endoscope can be positioned in the esophagus during VATS to help identify the ligamentum (**Fig. 12**). Once the esophagus and ligamentum are identified, right-angle or curved Kelly forceps are used to dissect the ligamentum free from the esophagus (**Fig. 13**). A 5-mm bipolar vessel-sealing device is placed in the third port and used to seal and divide the ligamentum. Residual constriction can be evaluated with a flexible endoscope or by placing a Foley catheter in the esophagus and distending the balloon while retracting the balloon across the constricted region.

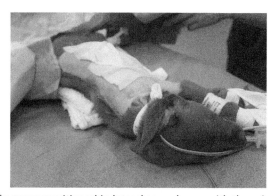

Fig. 11. Image of a puppy positioned in lateral recumbency with the spine slightly elevated before VATS ligamentum arteriosum ligation and division.

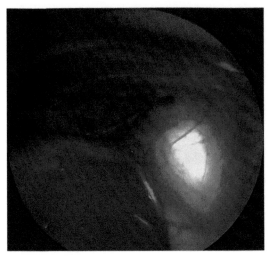

Fig. 12. Intraoperative image of the esophageal endoscope light demonstrating the location of the esophageal constriction.

Any remaining fibers should be excised to allow complete relief of the esophageal constriction.

PULMONARY NEOPLASIA

Video-assisted lung lobectomy is indicated for primary and metastatic pulmonary lesions.[21,22] Although early experience suggested that lesions away from the hilus of the left caudal lung lobe were most ideal for VATS lung lobectomy, a recent study has demonstrated feasibility in most lung lobes provided mass lesions are less than 8 cm in diameter or less than 150 cm^3 in dogs greater than 30 kg.[22]

Video-assisted lung lobectomy has been described.[21–23] The use of one-lung ventilation (OLV) is recommended during VATS lung resection to improve visibility and to facilitate application of the stapling device to the collapsed lung.[21,22] Identification of surgical margins is challenging and tracheobronchial lymphadenectomy and

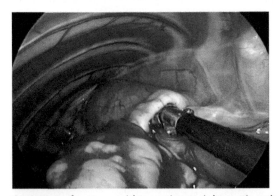

Fig. 13. Intraoperative image of a puppy with a persistent right aortic arch and left ligamentum undergoing ligamentum ligation and division. (*Courtesy of* Dr Eric Monnet, Colorado State University, Fort Collins, CO.)

histopathology is recommended to better assess prognosis and the need for adjunctive treatment in dogs with lung tumors.[22,24,25]

Recently, near-infrared field fluorescent (NIRF) technology has been investigated for pulmonary neoplasia VATS applications experimentally.[26] NIRF allows for activation of cancer cells in tissues, such as the pleura and lung. NIRF is considered a *smart* or *specific* form of fluorescent imaging, which creates a significant visible tumor-to-background ratio. The increased visible distinction between neoplastic and normal tissue, in addition to the superior illumination and visualization provided by VATS, seems to facilitate intraoperative assessment of surgical margins and sentinel lymph node assessment (**Figs. 14** and **15**). Although no literature on VATS applications of NIRF currently exists in veterinary surgery, early evidence supports the use of NIRF technology in this application and future study is indicated.[26–28]

The value of tracheobronchial lymphadenectomy and histopathology has been established.[24] Consequently, the surgeon performing VATS lung lobectomy must have a plan to assess these lymph nodes to better treat and prognosticate their patients. Tracheobronchial lymphadenectomy is feasible in dogs and has recently been described in clinical and experimental settings.[22,29] Tracheobronchial lymphadenectomy is performed in lateral recumbency and OLV is recommended to facilitate visualization of the tracheobronchial lymph nodes (TBLN) and to impart increased safety during the dissection.[22,29] The left TBLNs are approached from the left side and the central and right TBLNs are approached from the right.[29]

The affected hemithorax is clipped completely from dorsal to ventral across midline and from the caudal cervical region to the cranial abdomen. Dogs are positioned in lateral recumbency with the dorsal spine slightly elevated. Once the dog is positioned, OLV is induced using a double-lumen endobronchial tube (**Fig. 16**) or an endobronchial blocker.[21,22,29,30] Three to four 5.5- and/or 11.5-mm cannulas are typically required for VATS lung lobectomy. For access to cranial lung lobes, cannulas are placed in triangulating fashion along the ninth and tenth intercostal spaces (**Fig. 17**). For caudal and middle lobes, cannulas are placed along the third, fourth, or fifth intercostal spaces. For caudal lung lobectomy, the pulmonary-diaphragmatic ligament must be divided before lobectomy. A blunt palpation probe is helpful to elevate and

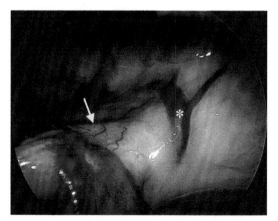

Fig. 14. Intraoperative image of a dog with a lung tumor before tracheobronchial lymphadenectomy. The asterisk shows the azygous vein and the arrow shows the location of the TBLN. (*Courtesy of* Dr Michelle Steffey, University of California Davis, Davis, CA.)

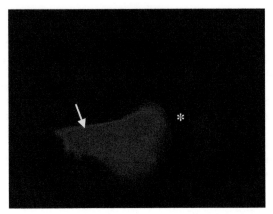

Fig. 15. Intraoperative image of the same dog from **Fig. 14** following administration of indocyanine green and visualization with NIRF. The asterisk shows the azygous vein and the arrow shows the location of the TBLN. (*Courtesy of* Dr Michelle Steffey.)

evaluate the parietal and visceral pulmonary surfaces (**Fig. 18**). Once the affected lung has been isolated, a 45- or 60-mm endoscopic stapler is inserted via one of the 11.5-mm cannulas or an additional cannula can be placed to allow unrestrained access to the pulmonary hilus (**Fig. 19**). For complete lung lobectomy, the stapler is

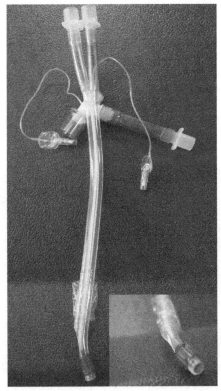

Fig. 16. Double-lumen endobronchial tube. The inset shows the angled bronchial portion of the tube and the Murphey eye from the endotracheal region.

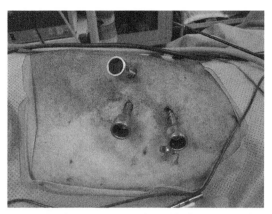

Fig. 17. Intraoperative image showing cannula location for a dog undergoing VATS caudal-lung lobectomy. (*Courtesy of* Dr Phil Mayhew, University of California Davis, Davis, CA.)

directed to the most proximal aspect of the pulmonary hilus before deploying the staples (**Fig. 20**). The lung lobe should be placed in an endoscopic tissue retrieval bag before extraction from the thorax to reduce the risk of neoplastic port site implantation.

TBLN excision can be performed by incising the pleura around the local TBLN followed by a combination of blunt dissection using right-angle Kelly forceps and vessel-sealing tissue dividing instruments. The TBLNs are immediately adjacent to the pulmonary artery and vein so caution should be exercised during the dissection.

Recently, a video-assisted, extracorporeal method for lung lobectomy or thoracoscopic-assisted pulmonary surgery was described in three cats and eight dogs.[31] This hybrid approach to lung lobectomy offers a minimally invasive alternative to open thoracotomy but at the same time eliminates the requirement for OLV and intracorporeal stapling.[31] Patients are prepared similarly to that described for VATS lung lobectomy.

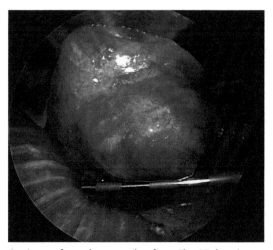

Fig. 18. Intraoperative image from the same dog from **Fig. 17** showing atraumatic palpation and manipulation of the mass with a blunt palpation probe. (*Courtesy of* Dr Phil Mayhew.)

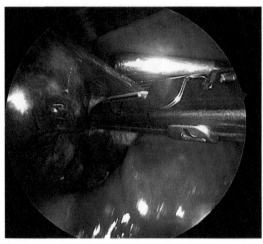

Fig. 19. Intraoperative image from the same dog with a 60-mm endoscopic stapler applied to the hilus of the caudal lung lobe. (*Courtesy of* Dr Phil Mayhew.)

Patients are positioned in lateral recumbency with the diseased hemithorax upper-most. A 5.5-mm cannula with a 5-mm 30° telescope is placed initially for exploration of the hemithorax and identification of the diseased lung. The intercostal location of the telescope cannula may vary but it is recommended that cranial lobes be explored from the 9th to 12th intercostal spaces and caudal lobes from the fourth to sixth intercostal spaces. Once the affected lobe is identified, a miniature extraction thoracotomy is made over the hilus of the lobe and a wound retractor placed to distract the intercostal wound (**Fig. 21**). The affected lobe is grasped with Babcock forceps or the surgeon's finger under intracorporeal visualization and elevated via the extraction wound (**Fig. 22**). Either partial or complete lung lobectomy is then performed using endo-scopic or traditional stapling devices (**Fig. 23**). TBLNs should be evaluated before

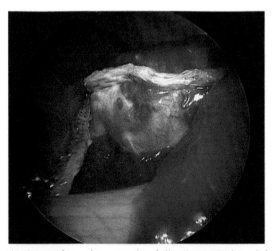

Fig. 20. Intraoperative image from the same dog following VATS lung lobectomy. (*Courtesy of* Dr Phil Mayhew.)

lobectomy and extirpation performed if medically indicated. The miniature thoracotomy and cannula incisions are closed routinely following placement of an indwelling chest tube. In this report, median surgery time and time to discharge were 90 minutes and 3 days, respectively. No significant complications were reported and all patients survived to hospital discharge.[31]

SPONTANEOUS PNEUMOTHORAX

VATS treatment of spontaneous pneumothorax in dogs has been described in 3 and 12 dogs.[32,33] In the original case report, three dogs were treated successfully without complications and all had a good outcome.[32] More recently, in a report of 12 dogs with spontaneous pneumothorax and pulmonary blebs and bullae, a rate of conversion to thoracotomy of 50% to 60% was reported because of inability to consistently identify active pulmonary leaks.[33] In this study adhesions and type 1 pulmonary lesions were thought to be the cause of inability to identify active leaks in several dogs. In one dog an adhesion in the dorsal and cranial aspect of the left cranial lobe was identified following median sternotomy. The lobe was found to leak only after conversion and disruption of the adhesion. In another dog, a missed bulla was identified at postmortem examination after failure of resolution of the pneumothorax. This case was not converted to median sternotomy. The conclusions and recommendations from this report were to anticipate a high rate of conversion and to convert all cases of spontaneous pneumothorax if an explanatory lesion was not identified and treated during VATS. Finally, as is seen in human surgery, a VATS approach to spontaneous pneumothorax may be associated with a higher rate of recurrence.[33]

Exploratory and Partial Lung Lobectomy

Dogs are positioned in dorsal recumbency and are tilted about 15° to the right (**Fig. 24**) and left for evaluation of individual hemithoraces. Individual lung lobes are evaluated on the pleural and parietal surfaces. Following initial evaluation, each lobe is submerged in saline and a positive-pressure breath hold initiated (**Fig. 25**). In instances where significant expansion of the lung lobes is necessary to elicit a leak, obliteration of working room occurs, which prevents assessment of the pleural surfaces.[33] This is

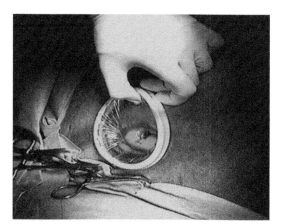

Fig. 21. Creation of a miniature thoracotomy and positioning of a surgical wound retractor over the hilus of the lung during thoracoscopic-assisted pulmonary surgery (TAPS). (*Courtesy of* Dr Jeff Runge, University of Pennsylvania, Philadelphia, PA.)

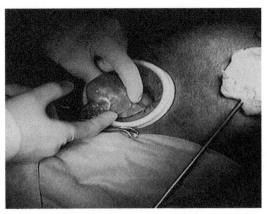

Fig. 22. Elevation of the lung to be removed by the surgeon's finger during TAPS. (*Courtesy of* Dr Jeff Runge.)

particularly true of type 1 pulmonary lesions and the author of this article has found these lesions exceptionally difficult to identify with a VATS approach. Consequently, if an active leak or lesion is not identified, conversion to median sternotomy is strongly recommended.[33]

If an active leaking lesion is identified during surgery, then partial or complete lung lobectomy can be performed (**Fig. 26**). For lesions in the middle to dorsal aspect of the lung lobe where a larger or complete lobectomy is necessary, the dog can be tilted and additional ports placed more dorsally to facilitate application of the endoscopic stapler. A 60-mm endoscopic stapler is recommended in most cases, and initiation of OLV is helpful during application of the endoscopic stapler. Saline can be infused on the staple line, and a breath hold maneuver performed to check for leaks (**Fig. 27**).

For mid to apical lesions in which a partial lobectomy is indicated, an articulated endoscopic stapler can usually be applied via one of the ventral intercostal ports. Again, initiation of OLV is useful to facilitate application of the endoscopic stapling device.

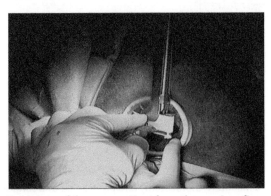

Fig. 23. Intraoperative image of the same patient from the previous figures showing stapled lung lobectomy during TAPS. (*Courtesy of* Dr Jeff Runge.)

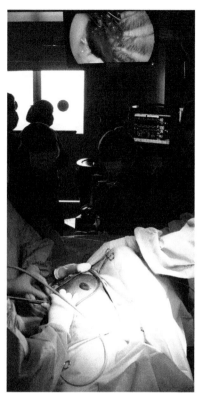

Fig. 24. Intraoperative image of a dog in dorsal recumbency being tilted to the right for VATS exploration and assessment of the left hemi-pleura.

The author of this article prefers to remove diseased lung from the thorax with an endoscopic retrieval bag because in some cases, bulla may result from neoplastic disease, which may not be diagnosed until histopathologic analysis has been completed.

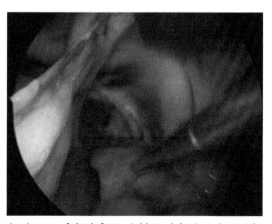

Fig. 25. Intraoperative image of the left cranial lung lobe in a dog with spontaneous pneumothorax being submerged in sterile saline to assess for pulmonary rupture.

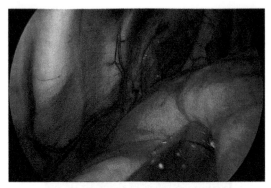

Fig. 26. Intraoperative image of a dog undergoing VATS partial lung lobectomy. Only the parietal pleural surface is shown but both surfaces are evaluated before partial lung lobectomy.

Following exploration and lung lobectomy, all port sites are closed routinely. Again, if an explanatory lesion or actively leaking lobe is not identified, conversion to median sternotomy is strongly recommended.

CHYLOTHORAX

Idiopathic chylothorax is a frustrating disease in dogs and cats and is often associated with recurrence or failure after initial therapy. Generally speaking, surgical treatment is the standard of care for idiopathic chylothorax in dogs and cats because medical therapy alone is unlikely to resolve the condition. A myriad of surgical treatments have been described and performed where the aims are ultimately to eliminate antegrade flow of chyle through the thoracic duct and/or to remove chylous effusion from the thorax. The most common procedures performed for cessation of chyle flow through the thoracic duct are thoracic duct ligation or embolization, cysterna chili ablation, and pericardectomy. Techniques used to remove fluid from the thorax include pleuroperitoneal shunt placement and thoracic omentalization. Success rates for resolution of chylous effusion following surgical intervention range from 80% to 100% in dogs and cats with most surgeons performing a combination of thoracic duct ligation,

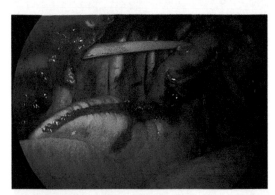

Fig. 27. Intraoperative image of the same dog from the previous figure following partial lobectomy. The catheter is being used to drip saline over the suture line to assess for leakage.

pericardectomy, and/or cysterna chili ablation.[34–38] Because access to multiple regions of the body is needed for these procedures, a video-assisted thoracic approach to the thoracic duct and pericardium may be of significance in dogs undergoing surgical treatment of idiopathic chylothorax. Two techniques have been described for VATS thoracic duct ligation and pericardectomy in dogs.[34,35] The original report used an intercostal VATS approach to the thoracic duct with the dog in sternal recumbency (**Fig. 28**), followed by alteration of the dog into dorsal recumbency for pericardectomy.[34] More recently, a similar approach was described but with the dogs in lateral recumbency for thoracic duct ligation followed by repositioning into dorsal recumbency for pericardectomy.[35]

Thoracic Duct Ligation

The entire thorax and abdomen are clipped and prepared aseptically for surgery. The dog is positioned in left lateral recumbency and the initial telescope portal is placed in the eighth or ninth intercostal space, approximately at the middle or dorsal third of the space (**Fig. 29**). Two instrument portals are then placed, one in the dorsal third of the ninth or tenth intercostal space and the other in the dorsal third of the seventh or eighth intercostal space. Five-millimeter cannulae are preferred for the telescope and dissecting instruments and at least one 11.5-mm cannula is required for the vessel-clip applicator. Once caudal mediastinal visualization has been accomplished, a miniature laparotomy is performed in the right lateral abdomen. A surgical wound retractor is used to retract the abdominal wall, and the ileocecocolic lymph nodes are isolated for injection of methylene blue. Less than 1 mL of a 1:1 solution of sterile saline to methylene blue is sufficient in most cases. Filling of the thoracic duct usually occurs within 5 to 10 minutes (**Fig. 30**). Once the thoracic duct is well visualized, dissection using a 5-mm vessel sealing device and 5-mm right-angle and Kelly forceps can commence. Dissection should be performed as caudal or near to the diaphragmatic crus as possible and all thoracic duct branches need to be identified and clipped (**Fig. 31**). Use of Harmonic shears for thoracic duct seal has been reported in a non-diseased, experimental canine model.[39] In this study, 50% of dogs were converted to an assisted miniature thoracotomy and 50% required resealing of the thoracic duct because of an inadequate initial seal. Ultimately, all six dogs experienced complete seal of the thoracic duct as confirmed by postprocedure lymphangiography

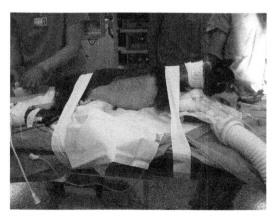

Fig. 28. Intraoperative image of a dog in sternal recumbency before VATS thoracic duct ligation. (*Courtesy of* Dr Phil Mayhew.)

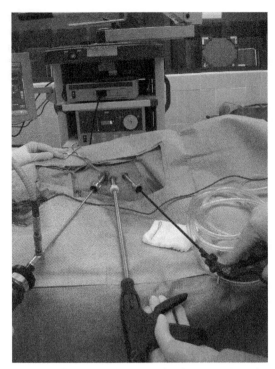

Fig. 29. Intraoperative view demonstrating cannula placement in a dog undergoing VATS thoracic duct ligation. (*Courtesy of* Dr Phil Mayhew.)

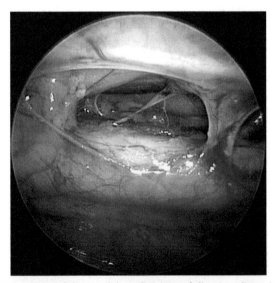

Fig. 30. Intraoperative view of the caudal mediastinum following dissection to the thoracic duct. Notice the thoracic duct is easily observed following administration of methylene blue. (*Courtesy of* Dr Phil Mayhew.)

and histopathology. Evaluation in dogs with naturally occurring disease is necessary before this can be recommended clinically.

It is strongly recommended that an intraoperative or postoperative lymphangiogram be performed to rule out continued thoracic duct patency following thoracic duct ligation. With the approach described by Mayhew and colleagues[35] this is easily accomplished immediately after thoracic duct ligation by reinjection of the ileocecocolic lymph nodes with iohexol under fluoroscopic visualization. The miniature laparotomy and portal sites are closed routinely.

Pericardectomy

If pericardectomy is to be performed, the dog can be repositioned into dorsal recumbency and a 4-cm apical pericardical window with pericardial fillet can be performed as previously described.[34] If a subphrenic pericardectomy is desired, then OLV has been recommended to improve visualization of the phrenic nerves during dissection.[40] Dissection of the pericardium is completed approximately 1 cm ventral and parallel to the phrenic nerves.

COMPLICATIONS

Complications include hemorrhage (great vessels, intercostal vessels, pericardium), pneumothorax (pulmonary pleura, missed bleb bullae), hypoxemia (V/Q mismatch, pleural space, pneumonia), and port site metastasis.

POSTOPERATIVE CARE

Thoracostomy drains are recommended following VATS (**Fig. 32**). Intrapleural and intercostal bupivicaine is administered for local analgesia. Intravenous opioids are administered for at least 24 hours postoperatively.

OUTCOMES
Pericardectomy and Pericardial Window

Median disease free interval (DFI) for dogs with idiopathic pericardial effusion treated by VATS pericardial window was 11.6 months and was significantly worse than dogs treated by subtotal pericardectomy (median DFI not reached) in one recent study.[2] However, dogs with a neoplastic cause for their pericardial effusion experienced a similar DFI

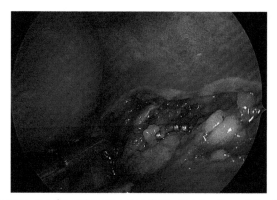

Fig. 31. Intraoperative view from the same dog following ligation of the thoracic duct with vessel clips. (*Courtesy of* Dr Phil Mayhew.)

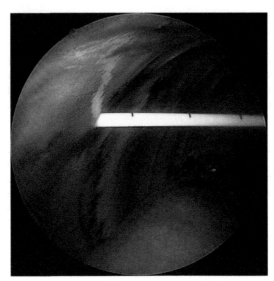

Fig. 32. Intraoperative image of a dog following a VATS procedure with a narrow chest tube placed.

if treated with a pericardial window (median DFI, 2.7 months) or a subtotal pericardectomy (median DFI, 3.8 months).

Similarly, median survival time (MST) for dogs with idiopathic pericardial effusion treated by VATS pericardial window was 13.1 months and was significantly worse than dogs treated by subtotal pericardectomy (MST not reached).[2] However, dogs with a neoplastic cause for their pericardial effusion experienced a similar MST if treated with a pericardial window (MST, 2.7 months) or a subtotal pericardectomy (MST, 4.0 months).

The 1-, 2-, and 3-year survival rates for dogs with an idiopathic pericardial effusion undergoing VATS pericardial window was 58%, 35%, and 35%, respectively. One-year survival for dogs with a neoplastic effusion undergoing VATS pericardial window was 9%.[2]

Cranial Mediastinal Mass Extirpation

CMM extirpation is an excellent application for VATS in select dogs. A conversion frequency of 10% has been reported but careful patient selection and proficiency with VATS will likely reduce the incidence of conversion.

Survival in dogs with a noninvasive thymoma undergoing VATS thymectomy was 100% in a recent study. In this same report, dogs with a thymoma and paraneoplastic myasthenia gravis with megaesophagus had an MST of only 20 days following successful VATS thymectomy.[16] Most of these dogs died of complications related to myasthenia gravis and megaesophagus (eg, aspiration pneumonia).

Left Ligamentum Division

Outcome is good to excellent in most dogs.[18–20]

Lung Lobectomy: Neoplasia

Although conversion to thoracotomy has been reported in up to 44% of dogs undergoing VATS lung lobectomy, a recent report has demonstrated a much lower rate (9%), which is likely the result of improved case selection and progressive experience with VATS lung lobectomy.[21,22] The reported median surgery times for VATS lung lobectomy are 108 and 120 minutes.[21,22] Clinical outcome is equivalent to dogs undergoing lung lobectomy via thoracotomy.[22] Survival is ultimately related to the underlying disease process as indicated by histopathology.

Pulmonary Exploratory and Partial Lung Lobectomy–Spontaneous Pneumothorax

Complete pleural exploratory and detection of pulmonary ruptures is challenging with a VATS approach in some cases. Recently, conversion to median sternotomy was required in 58% of dogs with spontaneous pneumothorax although conversion was not necessary in another report of three dogs with spontaneous pneumothorax.[32] Although clinical outcome may be good with a VATS approach to spontaneous pneumothorax in some dogs, only 50% of dogs treated with VATS without conversion experienced a successful clinical outcome. In contrast, 83% of dogs that underwent conversion to median sternotomy had a successful outcome.[33]

Thoracic Duct Ligation and Pericardectomy

Conversion to thoracotomy was not required in any dogs undergoing thoracic duct ligation for idiopathic chylothorax in two recent studies. Resolution of chylous effusion occurred in six out of seven dogs with idiopathic chylothorax and resolution of clinical signs occurred in six out of six dogs with a median follow-up time of 39 months, range 19 to 60 months in two separate studies.[34,35]

SUMMARY

The indications and applications for VATS are evolving constantly in veterinary surgery as more and more clients and surgeons are recognizing the benefits of reduced tissue trauma, less postoperative pain, and quicker recovery in their animals. As technology and experience continue to progress, this trend is sure to continue. Because specialized training and experience is a requirement and because VATS is associated with prolonged surgical times and certain limitations, prospective inquiries are indicated to better determine the relative benefits and possible limitations of VATS compared with traditional thoracotomy and sternotomy.

REFERENCES

1. Berg RJ, Wingfield WE. Pericardial effusion in the dog: a review of 42 cases. J Am Anim Hosp Assoc 1984;20:721–30.
2. Case JB, Maxwell M, Aman A, et al. Outcome evaluation of a thoracoscopic pericardial window procedure or subtotal pericardectomy via thoracotomy for the treatment of pericardial effusion in dogs. J Am Vet Med Assoc 2013;4:493–8.
3. Jackson J, Richter KP, Launder DP. Thoracoscopic partial pericardectomy in 13 dogs. J Vet Intern Med 1999;6:529–33.
4. Walsh PJ, Remedios AM, Ferguson JF, et al. Thoracoscopic versus open partial pericardectomy in dogs: comparison of postoperative pain and morbidity. Vet Surg 1999;6:472–9.
5. Dupre GP, Corlouer JP, Bouvy B. Thoracoscopic pericardectomy performed without pulmonary exclusion in 9 dogs. Vet Surg 2001;1:21–7.
6. Ployart S, Libermann S, Doran I, et al. Thoracoscopic resection of right auricular masses in dogs: 9 cases (2003-2011). J Am Vet Med Assoc 2013;2:237–41.
7. Crumbaker DM, Rooney MB, Case JB. Thoracoscopic subtotal pericardiectomy and right atrial mass resection in a dog. J Am Vet Med Assoc 2010;5:551–4.

8. Skinner OT, Case JB, Ellison GW, et al. Pericardioscopic imaging findings in cadaveric dogs: comparison of an apical pericardial window and sub-phrenic pericardectomy. Vet Surg 2014;1:45–51.

9. Barbur L, Radlinsky MG, Cornell KK, et al. Pericardial window with pericardial fillet for the treatment of pericardial disease in dogs. Proceedings of the 11th Annual Meeting of the Veterinary Endoscopy Society. Florence (Italy), May 15–17, 2014.

10. Culp TN. Surgical treatment of thymic disease. In: Monnet E, editor. Eric monnet small animal soft tissue surgery. 1st edition. Oxford (United Kingdom): Wiley-Blackwell Publishing; 2013. p. 72–81.

11. Atwater SW, Powers BE, Park RD, et al. Thymoma in dogs: 23 cases (1980-1991). J Am Vet Med Assoc 1994;7:1007–13.

12. Robat CS, Cesario L, Gaeta R, et al. Clinical features, treatment options, and outcome in dogs with thymoma: 116 cases (1999-2010). J Am Vet Med Assoc 2013;10:1448–54.

13. Zitz JC, Birchard SJ, Couto GC, et al. Results of excision of thymoma in cats and dogs: 20 cases (1984-2005). J Am Vet Med Assoc 2008;8:1186–92.

14. Garneau MS, Price LL, Withrow SJ, et al. Perioperative mortality and long-term survival in 80 dogs and 32 cats undergoing excision of thymic epithelial tumors. Vet Surg 2015;44(5):557–64.

15. Mayhew PD, Friedberg JS. Video-assisted thoracoscopic resection of noninvasive thymomas using one-lung ventilation in two dogs. Vet Surg 2008;8:756–62.

16. MacIver M, Case JB, Monnet EL, et al. Video-assisted cranial mediastinal mass extirpation in 18 dogs. Proceedings of the 12th Annual Meeting of the Veterinary Endoscopy Society. Santa Barbara (CA), April 12–14, 2015.

17. Kreb IA, Lindsley S, Shaver S, et al. Short- and long-term outcome of dogs following surgical correction of a persistent right aortic arch. J Am Anim Hosp Assoc 2015;50(3):181–6.

18. Isakow K, Fowler D, Walsh P. Video-assisted thoracoscopic division of the ligamentum arteriosum in two dogs with persistent right aortic arch. J Am Vet Med Assoc 2000;9:1333–6.

19. MacPhail CM, Monnet E, Twedt DC. Thoracoscopic correction of persistent right aortic arch in a dog. J Am Anim Hosp Assoc 2001;6:577–81.

20. Nucci D, Hurst K, Monnet E. Proceedings of the 12th Annual Meeting of the Veterinary Endoscopy Society. Santa Barbara (CA), April 12–14, 2015.

21. Lansdowne JL, Monnet E, Twedt DC, et al. Thoracoscopic lung lobectomy for treatment of lung tumors in dogs. Vet Surg 2005;5:530–5.

22. Mayhew PD, Hunt GB, Steffey MA, et al. Evaluation of short-term outcome after lung lobectomy for resection of primary lung tumors via video-assisted thoracoscopic surgery or open thoracotomy in medium- to large-breed dogs. J Am Vet Med Assoc 2013;5:681–8.

23. Monnet E. Interventional thoracoscopy in small animals. Vet Clin North Am Small Anim Pract 2009;5:965–75.

24. McNeil EA, Ogilvie GK, Powers BE, et al. Evaluation of prognostic factors for dogs with primary lung tumors: 67 cases (1985-1992). J Am Vet Med Assoc 1997;211:1422–7.

25. Martano M, Boston S, Morello E, et al. Respiratory tract and thorax. In: Kudnig ST, Seguin B, editors. Veterinary surgical oncology. Chichester (United Kingdom): Wiley Blackwell; 2012. p. 300–14.

26. Figueiredo JL, Alencar H, Weissleder R, et al. Near infrared thoracoscopy of tumoral protease activity for improved detection of peripheral lung cancer. Int J Cancer 2006;118:2672–7.

27. Holt DE, Madajewski B, Schuming N, et al. Near-infrared imaging detects cancer intraoperatively in canine primary lung tumors. Proceedings of the ACVS Annual Meeting. San Diego (CA), October 16–18, 2014.

28. Ashitate Y, Tanaka E, Stockdale A, et al. Near-infrared fluorescence imaging of the thoracic duct anatomy and function in open surgery and video-assisted thoracic surgery. J Thorac Cardiovasc Surg 2011;1:31–8.

29. Steffey MA, Daniel L, Mayhew PD, et al. Video-assisted thoracoscopic extirpation of the tracheobronchial lymph nodes in dogs. Vet Surg 2015;44(Suppl 1):50–8.

30. Mayhew PD, Culp WT, Pascoe PJ, et al. Evaluation of blind thoracoscopic-assisted placement of three double-lumen endobronchial tube designs for one-lung ventilation in dogs. Vet Surg 2012;6:664–70.

31. Wormser C, Singhal S, Holt DE, et al. Thoracoscopic-assisted pulmonary surgery for partial and complete lung lobectomy in dogs and cats: 11 cases (2008-2013). J Am Vet Med Assoc 2014;9:1036–41.

32. Brissot HN, Dupre GP, Bouvy BM, et al. Thoracoscopic treatment of bullous emphysema in 3 dogs. Vet Surg 2003;6:524–9.

33. Case JB, Mayhew PD, Singh A. Evaluation of video-assisted thoracic surgery for treatment of spontaneous pneumothorax and pulmonary bullae in dogs. Vet Surg 2015;44(Suppl 1):31–8.

34. Allman DA, Radlinsky MG, Ralph AG, et al. Thoracoscopic thoracic duct ligation and thoracoscopic pericardectomy for treatment of chylothorax in dogs. Vet Surg 2010;1:21–7.

35. Mayhew PD, Culp WT, Mayhew KN, et al. Minimally invasive treatment of idiopathic chylothorax in dogs by thoracoscopic duct ligation and subphrenic pericardectomy: 6 cases (2007-2010). J Am Vet Med Assoc 2012;7:904–9.

36. McAnulty JF. Prospective comparison of cisterna chili ablation to pericardectomy for treatment occurring idiopathic chylothorax in the dog. Vet Surg 2011;8:926–34.

37. Staiger BA, Stanley BJ, McAnulty JF. Single paracostal approach to thoracic duct and cisterna chili: experimental study and case series. Vet Surg 2011;7:786–94.

38. Fossum TW, Mertens MM, Miller MW, et al. Thoracic duct ligation and pericardectomy for treatment of idiopathic chylothorax. J Vet Intern Med 2004;3:307–10.

39. Leasure CS, Ellison GW, Roberts JF, et al. Occlusion of the thoracic duct using ultrasonically activated shears in six dogs. Vet Surg 2011;7:802–10.

40. Mayhew KN, Mayhew PD, Sorrell-Raschi L, et al. Thoracoscopic subphrenic pericardectomy using double-lumen endobronchial intubation for alternating one-lung ventilation. Vet Surg 2009;8:961–6.

Advances in Otoscopy

MaryAnn G. Radlinsky, DVM, MS

KEYWORDS

- Otoscopy • Ear • Dog • Cat • Endoscopy • Otitis

KEY POINTS

- Video-otoscopy is a wonderful tool for the assessment, diagnosis, and treatment of otitis, which is common in small animal practice.
- The lighting, magnification, and ability to lavage and introduce instruments are greatly enhanced with video-otoscopy over hand-held otoscopes.
- Documentation for the medical record and client education are also beneficial, and owners may be more compliant with therapy if they can see the condition of the ear canal themselves.

EQUIPMENT

There are many video-otoscopes available to the practitioner including the wireless Firefly Digital Video Otoscope (Firefly Global, Belmont, MA), Digital MacroView Otoscope (Welch Allen, Skaneateles Falls, NY), and multiple types available by JEDMED (St. Louis, MO).[1] The video-otoscopes most commonly used in veterinary medicine include the Otoscope for the Small Animal Practice (Karl Storz, Goleta, CA) and Video Otoscope (Med Rx, Inc, Largo, FL). A typical video-otoscope for veterinary practice is 5-mm diameter and 8.5-cm long with a 5F catheter working channel (**Fig. 1**). There is a stopcock attachment that allows for irrigation and passage of many instruments, including a diode laser, through the operating channel (**Fig. 2**); it and the otoscope are autoclavable for sterilization between uses. A camera, xenon light source, and monitor are required, and an image capture unit is extremely helpful for recording still and video images. Many types of instruments are available and include biopsy forceps, grasping forceps, and ear curettes (**Fig. 3**). Specialized accessories include a polypectomy snare and myringotomy needle. An extremely helpful accessory is the OTEX Brush (Karl Storz Veterinary Endoscopy, Goleta, CA, USA) for removing secretions adhered to the wall of the external ear canal. An automated flushing and suction pump makes deep ear cleaning extremely efficient (**Fig. 4**).

The author has nothing to disclose.
Department of Small Animal Medicine and Surgery, College of Veterinary Medicine, The University of Georgia, 2200 College Station Road, Athens, GA 30602, USA
E-mail address: radlinsk@uga.edu

http://dx.doi.org/10.1016/j.cvsm.2015.08.006
0195-5616/16/$ – see front matter
vetsmall.theclinics.com

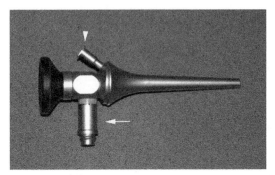

Fig. 1. Standard otoscope used for video-otoscopy. The black ring attaches to the camera adapter, the post (*arrow*) indicates the attachment of the light source, and the *arrowhead* indicates the port for instrument insertion or attachment site for irrigation.

Frequent use and use in the examination room with the client present are possible with most systems, and an all-in-one light source and image processor are available and can be used with the accessories and suction and irrigation pump (Tele Pack Vet X, Karl Storz).

The main benefits of video-otoscopy over traditional, hand-held otoscopes are the placement of the light at the tip of the endoscope, magnification, and projection of the image for viewing without the endoscopist's head being directly adjacent to the patient. An unimpeded view sans shadowing and entry of instruments immediately into the visual field improves the ability to use fine movements and manipulations within the tight space of the ear canal. Complete removal of cerumin, exudate, and foreign material is greatly enhanced by video-otoscopy. The risk of tympanic membrane rupture is minimized by the lighting and magnification provided with video-otoscopy; however, it cannot be eliminated, because the viewer is translating a three-dimensional experience onto a two-dimensional monitor, and the depth perception and ability to manipulate the instruments adjacent to the ear drum is not perfect and is a learned skill.

Care should be taken to avoid aggressive flushing of the ear canal during otoscopy and cleaning, and an egress of fluid is mandatory to avoid iatrogenic tympanic membrane rupture. Deeper examination of the ear is done through the tympanic membrane or its remnant in the case of a ruptured tympanum. A 2.7-mm endoscope is used to

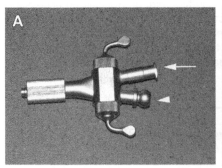
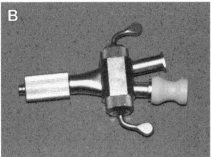

Fig. 2. (*A*) Attachment that allows concurrent use of irrigation (*arrow*) and instrumentation (*arrowhead*). (*B*) A grommet has been added to the instrument port to minimize fluid leakage during instrument use.

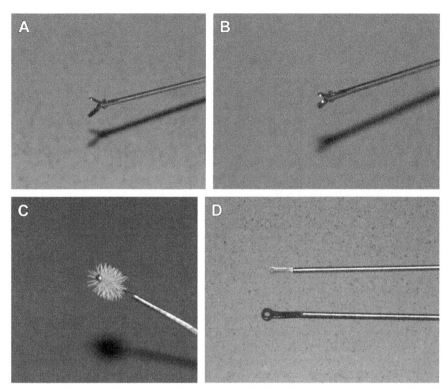

Fig. 3. (*A*) Flexible alligator grasping forceps. (*B*) Flexible biopsy forceps. (*C*) Flexible otoscopy brush. (*D*) Otoscopy currettes come in small and large sizes and can be angled to suit use.

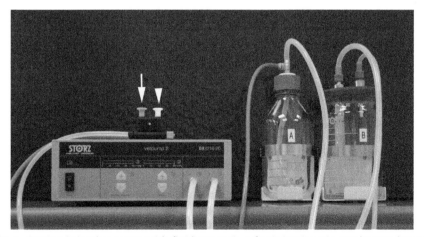

Fig. 4. Suction irrigation pump with fluid reservoir A for irrigation via one button (*arrow*) and aspiration via the other button (*arrowhead*), which allows fluid to be collected into reservoir B. (*Courtesy of* KARL STORZ GmbH & Co, Goleta, CA; with permission.)

enter the middle ear, which should be done in the ventral aspect of the tympanic membrane or at its previous location to avoid trauma to the acoustic or vestibular window. This requires knowledge of the anatomy of the ear canal and where the tympanic membrane should be. The depth must be estimated, because exudate, hair, cerumin, or mass lesions can obscure the view of an intact or ruptured tympanic membrane. An examination sheath can be used with a 2.7-mm endoscope to protect it from trauma, but irrigation through the sheath is not possible. An arthroscopic sheath allows for irrigation but instruments must be passed adjacent to the endoscope for use, which is possible because the viewing angle is offset at 30°. If instrument passage through a channel is desired, the cystoscope, or operating, sheath is required, which allows the passage of 5F catheter instruments; however, the diameter of the sheath is 14.5F catheter or 4.83 mm. Alternatively a 9.5F catheter or 3.17-mm, working endoscope is available, which has a 3F catheter working channel and a port for fluid irrigation. Biopsy and grasping forceps can be used through the working channel.

ANATOMY

The ear consists of the pinnae, external auditory meatus (external ear canal), middle ear, and inner ear. The canine external ear canal is 5 to 10 cm long and 4 to 5 mm wide and begins at the tragus, antitragus, and antihelix. Most practitioners understand the vertical and horizontal portions require specific manipulation to straighten the ear canal for visualization of the tympanic membrane. The manipulation required is the result of these two parts of the external ear canal and their separation by a dorsal fold. It is also important to know that the terminal horizontal ear canal is surrounded by bone, which cannot be dilated or manipulated, meaning it cannot be penetrated by large-diameter otoscopes or otoscope cones and could result in bending and damage of a long, rigid endoscope.

The tympanic membrane separates the external ear canal and the middle ear. It is normally thin and translucent ventrally at the pars tensa. The pars flaccida is dorsally located and is opaque. It can be minimally visible to distended with air or fluid in the middle ear, making it appear masslike. The pars tensa is the most familiar part of the tympanic membrane, is the largest part of the tympanic membrane, and is most often damaged. A visible portion of the manubrium of the malleus is rather straight in the cat and curves rostrally in the dog. Blood vessels are visible on its surface.

The middle ear has separate portions. The auditory ossicles are located in the rostral portion of the tympanic cavity and lead to the rostromedially located auditory and vestibular windows. The osseous tympanic bulla is the large portion that holds the opening of the auditory tube in its medial aspect.

INDICATIONS FOR VIDEO-OTOSCOPY

Because ear disease is common in general practice, one could use video-otoscopy in every examination, even with annual examinations. Specific clinical signs of ear disease include aural pruritis, aural pain, head shaking, malodor and otic discharge, facial excoriations, and aural hematoma formation. Animals with ear disease or dermatologic conditions should undergo a complete and a focused history, general physical examination, otic examination and otoscopy, and dermatologic evaluation. The ears should be examined from the pinna to the tympanic membrane for redness, pain, swelling, firmness, hardness, and discharge. Palpation of the ear canals for pliability, comfort level, swelling, and shape should be done. Abnormalities include pain; redness; firm, noncompliant external ear canals; or thick and hard canals suggestive of calcification. Cranial nerves should be evaluated through examining facial symmetry and response and motion of the ears with stimulation of the external ear canal lumen. Abnormalities include alteration in the carriage of the oral commisures, palpebral fissures, third eyelids, and pupils. Evaluate the palpebral reflex, pupillary light reflex, and facial sensation (via stimulation of the vibrissae on the muzzle, medial aspect of the nares, and ear canal lumen) and watch for reaction (movement away from the stimulation and moving the ears and pinnae). Cranial nerve evaluation should include evaluating for vestibular signs (nystamus, strabismus, head tilt), facial nerve paralysis, and Horner syndrome.

OTOSCOPIC EXAMINATION

Otoscopic examination should start at a landmark that allows the otoscope to enter the external ear canal repeatedly and successfully: the intertragic incisure is that landmark (**Fig. 5**). Grasp the base of the pinna and retract the ear dorsally and slightly laterally. This helps to minimize the interference of the dorsal fold with advancing the otoscope. Once the dorsal fold is passed (**Fig. 6**), retract the pinnal laterally and ventrally to pass the otoscope down the horizontal canal to the tympanic membrane (**Fig. 7**). Note the amount of erythema, swelling, and discomfort and any accumulation of exudate or cerumin and the presence of foreign material, hair, or mass lesions (**Fig. 8**). Video-otoscopy allows for immediate digital still and video imaging, which can be maintained as part of the medical record. The appearance of both ears should be documented.

An initial examination should be done on the awake patient. Start with the normal or more normal ear to familiarize yourself with the normal anatomy and depth of the tympanic membrane. Proper restraint and taking care to maintain the otoscope centrally within the external ear canal and avoiding contact of the otoscope along the wall of the ear canal during the examination helps to minimize patient discomfort. Properly

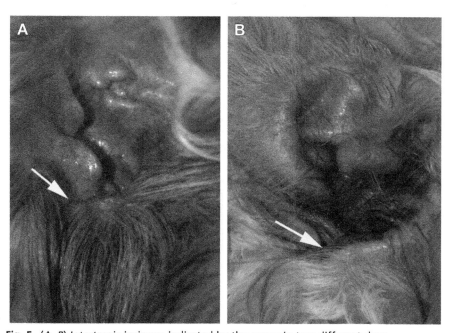

Fig. 5. (*A, B*) Intertragic incisures indicated by the *arrow* in two different dogs.

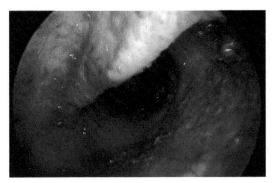

Fig. 6. Dorsal fold as seen during video-otoscopy.

restraining the head aids in the process. Place the palm of the hand on the dorsal aspect of the muzzle in dogs and direct the fingers downward on the sides of the maxilla with the thumb on the opposite side of the maxilla. Angle the head downward, which provides the best restraint against the most common reaction in dogs, which is to quickly and strongly elevate the muzzle during otoscopy. "Scraping" the otoscope along the wall of the ear canal happens when the lumen of the ear canal is not maintained in a central position within the field of view, and the wall of the canal is readily visible. Significant aural pain, cerumin, exudate, thickening, stenosis, or calcification of the ear canal may limit the ability to examine the ear canals in awake patients.

Significant exudate or cerumin, inflammation, pain, or stenosis may also require treatment before examining the entire external ear canal and tympanic membrane, and such treatment is best based on cytologic examination, which is beyond the scope of this article. Significant amounts of exudate or cerumin may require removal to allow for proper topical treatment of the external ear canal. General anesthesia with endotracheal intubation are required for deep ear cleaning, which requires significant flushing of the ear canal, thus warranting the endotracheal tube to minimize the risk of tracheal contamination with fluid that flows out of the external ear canal or via aspiration of fluid that traverses the auditory tube if the tympanic membrane is ruptured before or inadvertently during the procedure.

General anesthesia is indicated for examination of patients with the previously mentioned otic conditions and those with vestibular signs, Horner syndrome, otic foreign material, an abnormal tympanic membrane, and recurrent or chronic otitis. General anesthesia is also required for deep ear cleaning for the diagnosis and treatment of similar conditions as those listed previously. Place the patient in lateral

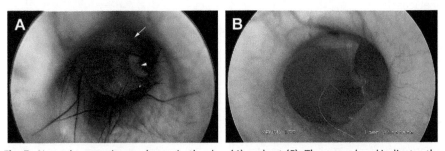

Fig. 7. Normal tympanic membrane in the dog (A) and cat (B). The *arrowhead* indicates the rostral aspect of the malleus and the *arrow* indicates the pars flaccida.

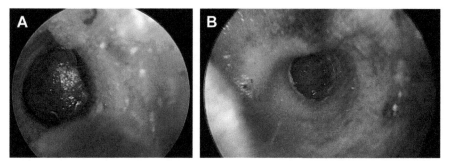

Fig. 8. Pathology of the ear. (*A*) Ceruminolith adjacent to the tympanic membrane in a dog. (*B*) Inflammatory polyp in a cat.

recumbency and stand at the patient's ventral aspect. This allows the image to maintain an orientation equal to that of hand-held otoscopy. Manipulation of the ear is also normal as for hand-held otoscopy. The otoscope and ear canal should be manipulated as described for examination in the awake patient. Document all portions of the ear canal and tympanic membrane with still or video images. Evaluate for the health of the canal and for foreign material and parasites. Document the state of the epithelium for erythema, exudate, ulceration, proliferation, stenosis, and mass lesions. Hair may be present in the normal ear canal, but loose hairs and large accumulation of hair may be abnormal; however, removal of normal hair is not typically done because it may result in epithelial inflammation. Damage to the epithelium may also predispose the patient to bacterial colonization and proliferation. Once the initial examination is done, samples should be taken for cytology and culture as necessary for the patient.

Deep ear cleaning can then be done if necessary to allow full examination of the external ear canal and tympanic membrane. Again, endoscopy of the normal or more normal ear should be done first to estimate the depth of the tympanic membrane to avoid iatrogenic rupture. If the tympanic membrane cannot be visualized, use sterile saline to clean the ear canal. A suction irrigation pump is incredibly helpful for this purpose and increases the efficiency of the procedure. A 5F polypropylene catheter should be cut to a length that is longer than the ear canal, which allows it to be cut shorter as needed should it become obstructed with cerumin or exudate. A hand-held set of buttons allows intermittent lavage and suction by the operator. A ceruminolytic safe for use with a ruptured tympanic membrane may be used. Ceruminolytics greatly decrease the time required for deep ear cleaning. They are typically rather greasy, so cover the opening of the external ear canal with a cotton ball after instillation, hold the pinna with a gauze sponge, and massage the ear canal after instillation for at least 3 minutes. Completely clear the ceruminolytic with saline lavage and repeat if necessary.

Exudate, ceruminolyths, and foreign material may require more manipulation for removal. Simply placing the polypropylene catheter deep to the material in question may allow it to passively flow out of the ear canal with the efflux of saline. It may also loosen the material enough to be removed with suction applied to the catheter, grasping forceps, or a cotton-tipped applicator. Remnant exudate or cerumin can also be removed using the OTEX brush. Material that does not occlude the lumen but adheres to the epithelium can be lavaged, and continuous infusion of saline by gravity can accompany use of the brush for such material. Simply rotating the brush during extraction of the otoscope and continuing visualization allows the remnant material to be extracted. Be certain to not pull the brush into the working channel of the otoscope because that would push the material off of the brush onto the endo-scope tip, into the working channel, and onto the ear canal lining. Ear curettes may also be of value for remnant material in the external ear canal. Similar to the brush, advance the curette and then retrieve it while trapping material against the epithelium; make sure to avoid excessive pressure on the epithelium that would cause trauma. Material located against the tympanic membrane can be manipulated with gentle lavage, suction applied to the catheter, or grasping forceps. Great care to avoid iatro-genic tympanic membrane rupture should be used.

The tympanic membrane should be thin and translucent, with the pars flaccida in a neutral position or not visible. The manubrium of the malleus should be readily visible as should the normal vasculature of the tympanic membrane. Changes to the tym-panic membrane include thickening, erythema, edema, and fluid seen behind the membrane. Images should be made and notations of the location of any rupture. A rupture should be strongly suspected if air bubbles are seen traveling up and out with the flow of saline during lavage. Bubbles may actually be seen eminating from the middle ear if a clear view of the tympanum is present. The size and length of the video-otoscope precludes entry into the middle ear and is helpful to gauge the lack of a tympanic membrane, but should not be the sole means of determining its pres-ence or absence. Palpation with the polypropylene catheter or a softer, red rubber catheter is used to determine whether a structure is the tympanic membrane.[1] The softer catheter bends with gentle pressure against an intact tympanic membrane and advances without altered shape if a rupture is present.

ASSESSING THE TYMPANIC CAVITY

If the tympanic membrane is thickened, hyperemic, absent, or bulging or the malleus is not apparent, or there is visible fluid behind it or a mass affect, then the tympanic cavity should be assessed. Ideally, otoscopy is done in combination with computed tomography or MRI. Then the clinician knows if the tympanic cavity should be sampled or examined, which decreases the risk of introducing bacteria and/or hemorrhage, which could predispose to otitis media in cases with a normal middle ear. If the tym-panic membrane is absent, simply introduce the polypropylene catheter into the mid-dle ear, directing the catheter ventrally to avoid trauma to the ossicles or acoustic or vestibular windows. Collect fluid for culture and cytology. Specimens for culture and cytology can be obtained via endoscopic guided myringotomy. A spinal needle or 5F catheter polypropylene catheter can be used. Cut the end of a sterile polypropylene catheter at an angle to mimic that of a hypodermic needle and attach a 6- or 12-mL syringe to the catheter. Introduce the catheter through the ventral tympanic mem-brane, avoiding obvious blood vessels, and direct the catheter caudoventrally. Aspi-rate immediately on entering the tympanic cavity. If no fluid is obtained, saline can be gently infused into the tympanic bulla and aspirated.

TREATMENT OF THE TYMPANIC CAVITY

Fluid, exudate, cerumin, and other material should be removed from the middle ear. Mass lesions can also be debulked and sampled for histopathologic examination, which represents an advanced level of skill beyond that of normal video-otoscopy. The tympanic cavity can be lavaged to remove fluid, exudate, and cerumin through a ruptured tympanic membrane or with a 5F catheter polypropylene catheter intro-duced via myringotomy. Gentle instillation of saline followed by lavage is done with care, avoiding the dorsal and medial aspects of the middle ear. Do not use excessive pressure, because that alone could cause damage to the ossicles or the acoustic or vestibular windows and could lead to vestibular signs, facial nerve paresis or paralysis, Horner syndrome, or otitis interna. Owners should be warned of the potential complications; however, lavage of the tympanic cavity may be successful for treating otitis media and may be useful to avoid ventral bulla osteotomy.[2]

AFTERCARE

All lavage solution should be removed from the ear canal and tympanic cavity following video-otoscopy. Some clinicians treat the ear with topical therapy dictated by cytology before recovery from general anesthesia. Presumptive treatments should be implemented based on cytology, pending culture and susceptibility results when indicated. Systemic and topical therapy for otitis is beyond the scope of this article, but is started pending final results. Re-evatuation in 3 to 6 weeks should be done to monitor response to therapy and to evaluate for healing of the tympanic membrane, if rupture was present or if myringotomy was performed. Healing occurs in most cases with a 4-month period; however, severe damage to the germinal epithelium or blood supply can lead to permanent loss of the tympanic membrane.

SUMMARY

Video-otoscopy is a wonderful tool for the assessment, diagnosis, and treatment of otitis, which is common in small animal practice. The lighting, magnification, and ability to lavage and introduce instruments are greatly enhanced with video-otoscopy over hand-held otoscopes. Documentation for the medical record and client education are also beneficial, and owners may be more compliant with therapy if they can see the condition of the ear canal themselves. Lastly, owners can be shown the progress of their efforts on re-examination. Video-otoscopy can be used regularly during client visits and deep ear cleaning and assessment of the middle ear may be of great benefit in patient management.

REFERENCES

1. Angus JC, Campbell KL. Uses and indications for video-otoscopy in small animal practice. Vet Clin North Am Small Anim Pract 2001;31(4):809–28.
2. Palmeiro BS, Morris DO, Wiemelt SP, et al. Evaluation of outcome of otitis media after lavage of the tympanic bulla and long-term antimicrobial drug treatment in dogs: 44 cases (1998–2002). J Am Vet Med Assoc 2004;225(4):548–53.

Index

Note: Page numbers of article titles are in **boldface** type.

A

Anesthesia/anesthetics
    for endoscopy, **31–44**
        introduction, 31–32
        management of, 36
        monitoring of, 35–36
        pneumoperitoneum effects of, 32–33
        premedication, induction, and maintenance agents, 33–35
        preoperative preparation, 33
        recovery from, 41
    for laparoscopic surgery, 36–38
    for thoracoscopic surgery, 38–40
Automated suturing devices
    in laparoscopic surgery, 18–28
        blunt dissection probe, 20–21
        dissecting instruments, 18
        EndoStitch, 18
        energy-based devices, 22
        5 mm miniretractor, 21
        laparoscopic aspirator/lavage with monopolar hook, 21
        laparoscopic stapling, 25–28
        monopolar pencil electrode extensions, 21
        roticulating Maryland dissector, 19–20
        SILS Stitch, 18
        ultrasonic energy devices, 24–25
        vessel-sealing devices, 22–23

B

Bladder
    overactive
        botulinum-A toxin injection for, 132
Bladder masses
    benign
        endoscopic polypectomy for, 128–129
Bladder stone removal
    advances in, 126–128
        cystoscopic-guided stone basket retrieval, 126–127
        laser lithotripsy, 127
        PCCL, 127–128
Blunt dissection probe
    in laparoscopic surgery, 20–21

Vet Clin Small Anim 46 (2016) 181–191
http://dx.doi.org/10.1016/S0195-5616(15)00160-6
0195-5616/16/$ – see front matter © 2016 Elsevier Inc. All rights reserved.

Moving?

Make sure your subscription moves with you!

To notify us of your new address, find your **Clinics Account Number** (located on your mailing label above your name), and contact customer service at:

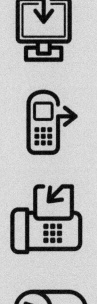

Email: journalscustomerservice-usa@elsevier.com

800-654-2452 (subscribers in the U.S. & Canada)
314-447-8871 (subscribers outside of the U.S. & Canada)

Fax number: 314-447-8029

Elsevier Health Sciences Division
Subscription Customer Service
3251 Riverport Lane
Maryland Heights, MO 63043

*To ensure uninterrupted delivery of your subscription, please notify us at least 4 weeks in advance of move.

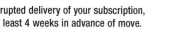
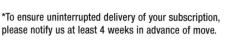